BTEC FIRST Health and Social Care

Val Michie

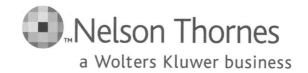

Nelson Thornes

a Wolters Kluwer business

Published in 2006 by:
Nelson Thornes Ltd
Delta Place
27 Bath Road
CHELTENHAM
GL53 7TH
United Kingdom

06 07 08 09 10 / 10 9 8 7 6 5 4 3 2 1

A catalogue record for this book is available from the British Library

ISBN 0 7487 8389 X

Cover photograph by Digital Vision
Illustrations by Angela Lumley and Pantek Arts Ltd
Page make-up by Pantek Arts Ltd, Maidstone, Kent
Printed and bound in Croatia by Zrinski

Contents

Introduction

Health and social care workers work with diverse groups of vulnerable people including children, young adults, elderly people and people with mental health problems and learning difficulties. They work in a variety of settings such as hospitals, care homes and people's own homes. Now is an exciting time to be a care worker because reforms are creating new jobs and flexible ways of working, and there is a huge amount of opportunity for career progression. If you are committed to working in care and enthusiastic about training and development, you can be assured of a challenging and rewarding career. The BTEC First Certificate or Diploma in Health and Social Care will get you off to a flying start by preparing you both for work in health or social care and for further study.

How do you use this book?

Covering all nine units of the new 2006 specification, this book has everything you need if you are studying BTEC First Certificate or Diploma in Health and Social Care. Simple to use and understand, it is designed to provide you with the knowledge and understanding you need to gain your qualification! We guide you step by step towards your qualification, through a range of features that are fully explained below.

Which units do you need to complete?

There are nine units available for BTEC First Health and Social Care. For the BTEC First Diploma in Health and Social Care you are required to complete two core units and four specialist units.

Core Units	Specialist Units
Unit 1 **Communication and Individual Rights within the Health and Social Care Sectors**	Unit 3 **Vocational Experience in a Health or Social Care Setting**
Unit 2 **Individual Needs within the Health and Social Care Sectors**	Unit 4 **Cultural Diversity in Health and Social Care**
	Unit 5 **Anatomy and Physiology for Health and Social Care**
	Unit 6 **Human Lifespan Development**
	Unit 7 **Creative and Therapeutic Activities in Health and Soical Care**
	Unit 8 **Health and Social Care Services**
	Unit 9 **The Impact of Diet on Health**

Is there anything else you need to do?

1. Talk to people who use health and social care services. Find out how they want to be cared for and what sort of qualities they would like to see in their care workers.
2. Talk to people who work in the health and social care industry. Find out what qualifications, skills and experience they needed to get their job and what their work involves.
3. Get as much experience as you can in the care industry and be aware of what your experiences teach you.
4. Take responsibility for learning about service users and the health and social care industry. In addition to completing all the work your teacher or tutor sets, ask questions and watch, read and listen to anything that will improve your knowledge and understanding.
5. Never be afraid to ask for help when you need it.

We hope you enjoy your BTEC course – Good Luck!

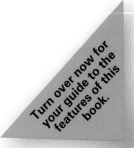

Turn over now for your guide to the features of this book.

Features of this book

Learning Objectives

At the beginning of each Unit there will be a bulleted list letting you know what material is going to be covered. They specifically relate to the learning objectives within the 2006 specification.

Grading Criteria

The table of Grading Criteria at the beginning of each unit identifies achievement levels of pass, merit and distinction, as stated in the specification.

To achieve a **pass**, you must be able to match each of the 'P' criteria in turn.

To achieve **merit** or **distinction**, you must increase the level of evidence that you use in your work, using the 'M' and 'D' columns as reference. For example, to achieve a distinction you must fulfil all the criteria in the pass, merit and distinction columns. Each of the criteria provides a specific page number for easy reference.

Activities

are designed to help you understand the topics through answering questions or undertaking research, and are either *Group* or *Individual* work. They are linked to the Grading Criteria by application of the D, P, and M categories.

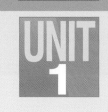

UNIT 1

Communication and Individual Rights within the Health and Social Care Sectors

This unit covers:
- Ways of promoting effective communication
- Barriers to effective communication
- Diversity and equality in society
- How the principles of the Care Value Base can be used to promote the rights of individuals and significant others.

To help develop relationships with service users, their colleagues, managers and others with whom they work, health and care workers need to have excellent communication skills. Good, supportive relationships are built on effective communication. However, misunderstandings can occur if there are difficulties in communicating. Because the role of health and care workers is to support the people they work with, it is important that they are able to recognise and prevent communication difficulties. It is also important that they develop an understanding of people's differences and how these differences affect work in a health or social care environment. This includes recognising people's rights, such as the right to be respected, to be treated equally and to not be discriminated against.

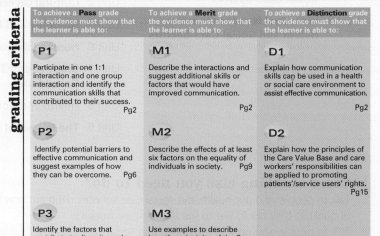

grading criteria

To achieve a **Pass** grade the evidence must show that the learner is able to:	To achieve a **Merit** grade the evidence must show that the learner is able to:	To achieve a **Distinction** grade the evidence must show that the learner is able to:
P1 Participate in one 1:1 interaction and one group interaction and identify the communication skills that contributed to their success. Pg2	**M1** Describe the interactions and suggest additional skills or factors that would have improved communication. Pg2	**D1** Explain how communication skills can be used in a health or social care environment to assist effective communication. Pg2
P2 Identify potential barriers to effective communication and suggest examples of how they can be overcome. Pg6	**M2** Describe the effects of at least six factors on the equality of individuals in society. Pg9	**D2** Explain how the principles of the Care Value Base and care workers' responsibilities can be applied to promoting patients'/service users' rights. Pg15
P3 Identify the factors that contribute to diversity and influence the equality of individuals in society. Pg9	**M3** Use examples to describe how the principles of the Care Value Base and care workers' responsibilities promote patients'/service users' rights. Pg15	

activity
GROUP WORK
(1.2)

D1

Health and care workers work with people who use alternative methods of communication.
- Find out about some of the alternative methods described above. You could contact charities such as those listed in the Information Bar below this Activity.
- Produce a display of your findings, which explains why alternative methods of communication are effective at helping service users.

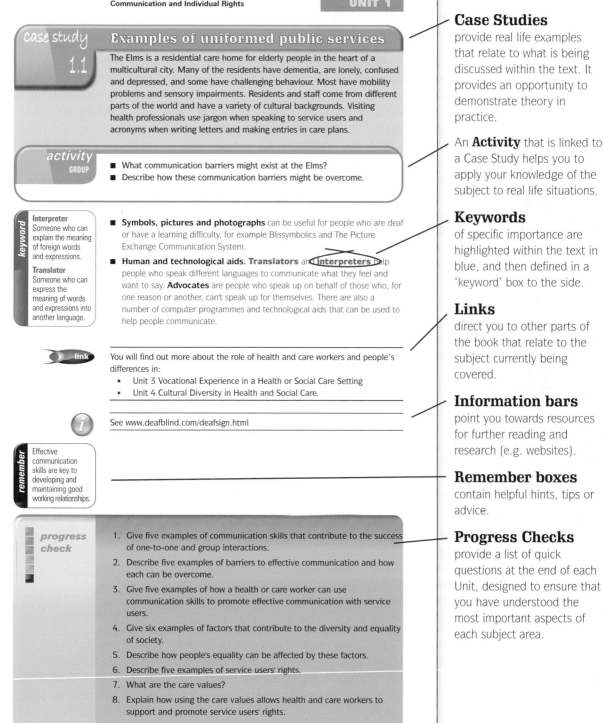

UNIT 1

case study 1.1
Examples of uniformed public services

The Elms is a residential care home for elderly people in the heart of a multicultural city. Many of the residents have dementia, are lonely, confused and depressed, and some have challenging behaviour. Most have mobility problems and sensory impairments. Residents and staff come from different parts of the world and have a variety of cultural backgrounds. Visiting health professionals use jargon when speaking to service users and acronyms when writing letters and making entries in care plans.

activity
GROUP

■ What communication barriers might exist at the Elms?
■ Describe how these communication barriers might be overcome.

keyword

Interpreter
Someone who can explain the meaning of foreign words and expressions.

Translator
Someone who can express the meaning of words and expressions into another language.

■ **Symbols, pictures and photographs** can be useful for people who are deaf or have a learning difficulty, for example Blissymbolics and The Picture Exchange Communication System.

■ **Human and technological aids. Translators** and **interpreters** help people who speak different languages to communicate what they feel and want to say. **Advocates** are people who speak up on behalf of those who, for one reason or another, can't speak up for themselves. There are also a number of computer programmes and technological aids that can be used to help people communicate.

link

You will find out more about the role of health and care workers and people's differences in:
• Unit 3 Vocational Experience in a Health or Social Care Setting
• Unit 4 Cultural Diversity in Health and Social Care.

i

See www.deafblind.com/deafsign.html

remember

Effective communication skills are key to developing and maintaining good working relationships.

progress check

1. Give five examples of communication skills that contribute to the success of one-to-one and group interactions.
2. Describe five examples of barriers to effective communication and how each can be overcome.
3. Give five examples of how a health or care worker can use communication skills to promote effective communication with service users.
4. Give six examples of factors that contribute to the diversity and equality of society.
5. Describe how people's equality can be affected by these factors.
6. Describe five examples of service users' rights.
7. What are the care values?
8. Explain how using the care values allows health and care workers to support and promote service users' rights.

Case Studies
provide real life examples that relate to what is being discussed within the text. It provides an opportunity to demonstrate theory in practice.

An **Activity** that is linked to a Case Study helps you to apply your knowledge of the subject to real life situations.

Keywords
of specific importance are highlighted within the text in blue, and then defined in a 'keyword' box to the side.

Links
direct you to other parts of the book that relate to the subject currently being covered.

Information bars
point you towards resources for further reading and research (e.g. websites).

Remember boxes
contain helpful hints, tips or advice.

Progress Checks
provide a list of quick questions at the end of each Unit, designed to ensure that you have understood the most important aspects of each subject area.

Acknowledgements

Crown copyright material is reproduced with the permission of the Controller of HMSO and the Queen's Printer for Scotland. Licence number: C2006009492.

Photograph credits:

David Buffington/Photodisc 67 (NT), p.31; Photodisc 14 (NT), p.32; Peter Casolino/Alamy, p.34; Dinodia Images/Alamy, p.36; Corbis V94 (NT), p.42, p.43; Image State Royalty Free/ Alamy, p.61; Image Source/Alamy, p.62; Image Source/Alamy, p.71 (left); fStop/Alamy, p.71 (top right); David R. Frazier Photolibrary/Alamy, p.71 (bottom right); Steven Allen/Brand X RW (NT), p.84 (top left and bottom right); Corel 750 (NT), p.84 (top right); C Sherburne/Photodisc 32 (NT), p.84 (bottom left); T O'Keefe/Photodisc 32 (NT), p.84 (bottom middle); Digital Stock 11 (NT), p.85; Corel 511 (NT), p.89 (top left); Steve Allen/Brand X RW (NT), p.89 (top right and bottom left); Digital Stock 11 (NT), p.89 (bottom right); BSIP, Edwige/Science Photo Library, p.119; Photofusion/Alamy, p.120; Custom Medical Stock Photo/Science Photo Library, p.121; Custom Medical Stock Photo/Alamy, p.123 (left); Mark Baigent/Alamy, p.123 (middle); Ian Hooton/Science Photo Library, p.123 (right); Ryan McVay/Photodisc 76 (NT), p.129 (left); Bananastock T (NT), p.129 (bottom left); Image 100/Alamy, p.129 (bottom middle); Bubbles/Angela Hampton, p.129 (right); Digital Vision TT (NT), p.132; Imageshop/Alamy, p.136 (left); bildagentur-online/begsteiger/Alamy, p.136 (right); Photodisc 63 (NT), p.138; Dynamic Graphics Photis/Alamy, p.152; Keith Brofsky/Photodisc 40 (NT), p.153; Julie Frazier/Photodisc 67 (NT), p.154; Gaetano Images/Alamy RF (NT), p.155; Keith Brofsky/Photodisc 59 (NT), p.160; Tina Manley/Alamy, p.161; Keith Brofsky/Photodisc 40 (NT), p.174 (left and middle); Photodisc 59 (NT), p.174 (right); Bananastock LT (NT), p.176; Keith Brofsky/Photodisc 59 (NT), p.178; Garry Watson/ Science Photo Library, p.184; Keith Brofsky/Photodisc 40 (NT), p.187; Janine Wiedel Photolibrary/Alamy, p.188 (left); Keith Brofsky/Photodisc 40 (NT), p.188 (right); Photofusion Picture Library/Alamy, p.200; Ryan McVay/Photodisc 71 (NT), p.202; Dr P. Marazzi/Science Photo Library, p.204 (left); Andy Crump, Tdr, Who/Science Photo Library, p.204 (right); Holt Studios/Alamy, p.211 (top left); Tim Graham/Alamy, p.211 (top right); Digital Vision 5 (NT), p.211 (bottom left); Corel 103 (NT), p.211 (bottom right).

All other photos by Martin Sookias.

I would like to thank all my friends, relatives, colleagues and other professionals whose help and support enabled me to write this book. In particular I would like to acknowledge:

Bubbles Higgins, Mary Michie and Rae Ellacott, for sharing with me their experiences of being cared for. Layla Baker, Angelo Veretto, Judy Cohen and Janis Morris, for their expert technical advice and guidance. Helen Broadfield, Jess Ward, Doug Forbes and Vanessa Thompson at Nelson Thornes, for all of their hard work.

Val Michie

Communication and Individual Rights within the Health and Social Care Sectors

This unit covers:

- ways of promoting effective communication
- barriers to effective communication
- diversity and equality in society
- how the principles of the Care Value Base can be used to promote the rights of individuals and significant others.

To help develop relationships with service users, their colleagues, managers and others with whom they work, health and care workers need to have excellent communication skills. Good, supportive relationships are built on effective communication. However, misunderstandings can occur if there are difficulties in communicating. Because the role of health and care workers is to support the people they work with, it is important that they are able to recognise and prevent communication difficulties. It is also important that they develop an understanding of people's differences and how these differences affect work in a health or social care environment. This includes recognising people's rights, such as the right to be respected, to be treated equally and to not be discriminated against.

<table>
<tr><td rowspan="2" style="writing-mode: vertical-lr">grading criteria</td><td>To achieve a Pass grade the evidence must show that the learner is able to:</td><td>To achieve a Merit grade the evidence must show that the learner is able to:</td><td>To achieve a Distinction grade the evidence must show that the learner is able to:</td></tr>
<tr><td>P1

participate in one 1:1 interaction and one group interaction and identify the communication skills that contributed to their success
Pg 6</td><td>M1

describe the interactions and suggest additional skills or factors that would have improved communication
Pg 6</td><td>D1

explain how communication skills can be used in a health or social care environment to assist effective communication
Pgs 8, 9</td></tr>
</table>

grading criteria

To achieve a **Pass** grade the evidence must show that the learner is able to:	To achieve a **Merit** grade the evidence must show that the learner is able to:	To achieve a **Distinction** grade the evidence must show that the learner is able to:
P2 identify potential barriers to effective communication and suggest examples of how they can be overcome Pg 13	**M2** describe the effects of at least six factors on the equality of individuals in society Pg 21	**D2** explain how the principles of the Care Value Base and care workers' responsibilities can be applied to promoting patients'/service users' rights Pg 26
P3 identify the factors that contribute to diversity and influence the equality of individuals in society Pg 17	**M3** use examples to describe how the principles of the Care Value Base and care workers' responsibilities promote patients'/service users' rights Pg 26	
P4 describe the rights of patients/service users Pg 23		
P5 identify the principles of the Care Value Base and care workers' responsibilities to patients/service users Pg 26		

Ways of Promoting Effective Communication

Health and social care workers need to be able to communicate effectively with **service users**. They need to understand how service users feel and what they want and need. They also need to be able to respond to service users' concerns and questions in ways that can be understood.

Health and social care workers also need to be able to communicate effectively with their colleagues, managers and other professionals. For example, they need to understand instructions and be able to pass on information which others can understand.

Understanding others, passing on information and making ourselves understood are key elements of the communication cycle.

The communication cycle

Imagine that you're with some friends, trying to decide where to go for a night out. You have an idea, for example 'Maybe the cinema … There's a good Brad Pitt film on at the moment.' Having an idea, thought or feeling is the beginning of a communication cycle.

Expressing an idea, thought or feeling and passing it on to others is the second stage of the communication cycle. In this situation you might say, 'Let's go to the cinema! They're showing Brad Pitt's latest film!'

For your friends to understand your idea, they have to be able to receive it and understand what you have said. Receiving someone's ideas, thoughts or feelings, and understanding what they mean or how they feel is the next stage in the communication cycle. In this situation, your enthusiasm to see Brad Pitt makes it quite plain to everyone what you want to do and how you feel!

The communication cycle continues when people respond with their own ideas, thoughts and feelings. In this situation, the next stage of the cycle is when your friends respond with what they think or feel about going to see the Brad Pitt film or offer up some ideas of their own.

All communication cycles have an end, for example when decisions are made or when time constraints mean that the communication has to finish. The communication cycle in this situation would end when everyone agrees about where to go for a night out.

Communication can be difficult when people have problems expressing themselves or if ideas, thoughts and feelings can't be understood. You will learn about communication difficulties shortly.

link

Links to Unit 3, page 66.

Figure 1.1

The communication cycle

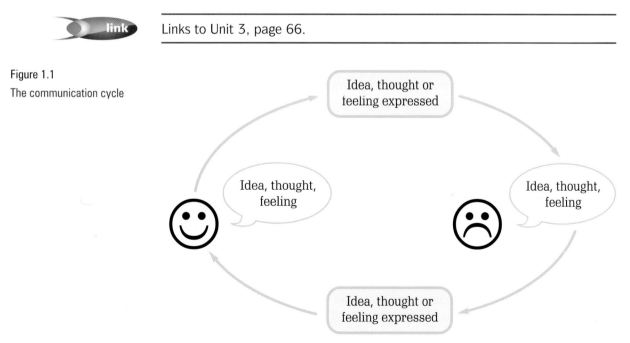

Forms of communication

One-to-one communications (interactions) are usually personal, private and specific to the people taking part. Group communications cover issues and topics that are of interest to everyone present.

Informal communications are relaxed and casual and allow people to be familiar with each other. Formal communications are more serious and official. Their main aim in health and care settings is to pass on important information to service users, colleagues and other health and care professionals.

Figure 1.2

Types of communication

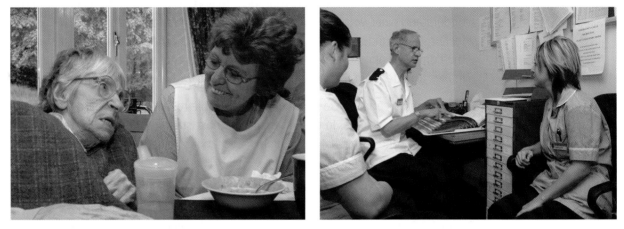

Verbal communication

Most communications have a verbal and a non-verbal aspect. Verbal communication is communication that uses speech. We use verbal communication to:

- tell other people how we feel and what we want
- find out things by asking questions
- pass on information and give directions.

Health and care workers need to use verbal communication effectively to encourage service users to communicate and to make themselves understood.

Figure 1.3

Effective use of verbal communication

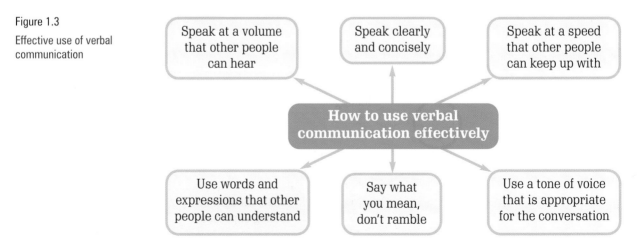

Speak at a volume that other people can hear

Speak clearly and concisely

Speak at a speed that other people can keep up with

How to use verbal communication effectively

Use words and expressions that other people can understand

Say what you mean, don't ramble

Use a tone of voice that is appropriate for the conversation

Non-verbal communciation

Non-verbal communication or body language is communication that doesn't use speech. We use it to show our feelings and our understanding of how other people feel.

- Facial expressions, e.g. frowns and smiles, tell other people how we feel. Using the same facial expression as the person talking to us shows that we understand how he or she feels.

Figure 1.4

Facial expressions can reveal how you feel

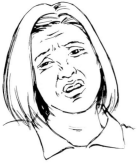
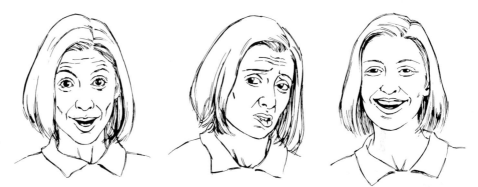

- Eye contact and body posture: a lack of eye contact and a bent posture can be signs of shyness and pain. Long periods of eye contact and a stiff posture can mean discomfort and frustration. Looking at someone and turning towards them shows we're interested in them.

- Body movements and gestures: repeated movements can be a sign of nervousness. Head nods can show interest in what is being said. Rubbing an area of the body can indicate pain but touching someone else can show concern for them.

Health and care workers need to use body language effectively to encourage service users to communicate and to make themselves understood.

Figure 1.5

Effective use of non-verbal communication

> Maintain an alert but comfortable posture

> Use facial expressions, eye contact and body movements that are appropriate and show interest

How to use non-verbal communication effectively

> Use touch if appropriate. Not everyone is comfortable with being touched, and others don't like their 'personal space' to be invaded. Be aware of people's views and preferences and only use touch if it is welcomed

To understand fully what service users want, need and feel, health and care workers should develop the skill of **active listening**. Active listening means:

- not interrupting. Wait until there is a gap in the conversation before speaking.

- respecting silences. Silences give people time to think about what they want to say.

- 'reading between the lines' of what the person is saying by observing his or her body language, asking questions and saying things like 'Yes' and 'I see' now and then. This shows you're trying to understand and encourages the person to continue.

- repeating what you heard the person say but in more simple language. This shows you're really listening and gives the speaker a chance to check your understanding of what they have said.

- not giving advice or your opinion unless it's asked for.

---

activity
GROUP WORK
(1.1)

P1

M1

Take part in:

1. a one-to-one communication, e.g. with your tutor

2. a group communication, e.g. with a group of friends.

At the end of each communication, ask for feedback on your communication skills. Make a list of:

(a) the effective verbal, non-verbal and active listening skills that you used

(b) the verbal, non-verbal and active listening skills that you need to develop.

Not everybody can communicate using speech or body language and some people have hearing difficulties. However, these people can be helped to communicate in a variety of alternative ways.

- Sign languages are used by people who are deaf or have difficulty speaking. They include British Sign Language (BSL) and signing through touch.

---

www.deafblind.com

Aids to communication

- Symbols, pictures and photographs can be useful for people who are deaf or have a learning difficulty, for example Blissymbolics and the Picture Exchange Communication System.

- Writing: people who have a hearing impairment can be helped by having messages written down. Braille, Moon and the deafblind manual alphabet are useful for people with a visual impairment.

Figure 1.6

The standard manual alphabet

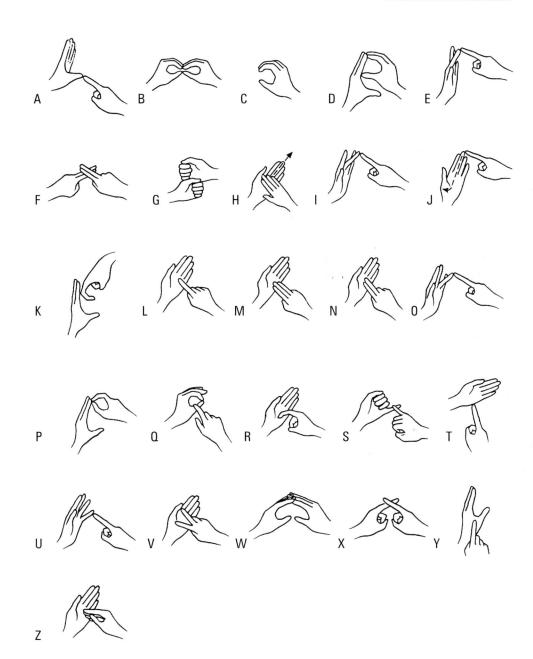

- People who have severe learning difficulties can be helped to communicate through the use of objects of reference. These are objects that are used daily and which have an obvious meaning, e.g. a picture of a plate.

- Human and technological aids: **interpreters** and **translators** help people who speak different languages to communicate what they feel and want to say. Advocates are people who speak up on behalf of those who, for one reason or another, can't speak up for themselves. There are also several computer programmes and technological aids that can be used to help people communicate.

activity
INDIVIDUAL WORK
(1.2)

D1

Health and care workers work with people who use alternative methods of communication.

(a) Find out about some of the alternative methods described above. You could contact charities such as those listed in the Information bar below this activity. These and other charities may have premises where you live. Visit them, telephone their national offices, or get in touch with them through their websites.

(b) Produce a display of your findings, which explains why alternative methods of communication are effective at helping service users.

Royal National Institute of the Blind www.rnib.org.uk
The Royal National Institute of the Deaf www.rnid.org.uk
Sense www.sense.org.uk
Scope www.scope.org.uk
The British Council of Disabled People www.bcodp.org.uk

Cultural differences

Cultural differences are based on differences in traditions, social customs, religions, age and sex, and they affect the way people communicate. Differences in the way people from different cultures communicate include variations in:

- body language. People from some cultures prefer much less 'personal space' around them than people from others. And some hand and foot gestures used in one part of the world can cause offence in another.

- the use of touch. People from some religions and age groups are not comfortable when touched by someone of the opposite sex.

- communicating pain. People from some cultures are very reserved about showing their feelings, whilst others are very public in communicating their distress.

- what they like to be called. People from some cultures are happy to be called by their first name, whilst others prefer to be addressed more formally, as Mr, Madam, etc.

- whom they are allowed to communicate with. People from some cultures will only communicate with someone of the same colour, sex, age and religion as themselves.

In order to communicate effectively with people from different cultures, health and care workers have a responsibility to communicate with them in ways with which they are most comfortable.

remember
Effective communication skills are key to developing and maintaining good working relationships and meeting the needs of service users.

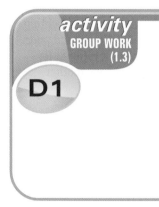

activity
GROUP WORK
(1.3)

D1

Health and care workers work with people who have a range of cultural backgrounds.

(a) Find out from two people who have different cultural backgrounds how their traditions, social customs, religions, age or sex affect the way they communicate.

(b) Produce an information sheet that explains how health and care workers should communicate with people from these two cultures in order that their health and care needs can be met.

Barriers to Effective Communication

If communication is to be effective, people must be able to express themselves clearly and to understand each other. Communication is ineffective when barriers prevent people expressing themselves or understanding others. This section describes some of the communication barriers that health and care workers meet in their day-to-day work and how they can help overcome them.

Sensory deprivation

People who have a sensory impairment have difficulty seeing or hearing.

People who are hard of hearing may not understand what they are told. And if they can't hear themselves very well, they can also have difficulty making themselves understood.

Figure 1.7

Overcoming barriers caused by hearing difficulties

> Make sure that the person wears their own hearing aid and that it is clean and in good working order

> Speak clearly and at a speed that the person can cope with

> Don't shout and keep background noise to a minimum. Shouting and background noise make it difficult for people to hear each other

How to help overcome communication barriers caused by hearing difficulties

> Use alternative forms of communication that are chosen by the person, e.g. sign language, lip reading, writing, pictures, **signers**

> Listen actively, using body language and eye contact to show you are interested

> Check that you and the person have understood each other by asking questions and repeating the message

keyword

Signer
Somebody who translates speech into signs that can be understood by people with a hearing impairment.

People with a sight impairment may find it difficult to see and understand writing, pictures and other people's body language.

Figure 1.8
Overcoming barriers caused
by sight impairment

> Make sure that the person wears their own glasses or contact lenses, that their glasses or contact lenses are clean and that the prescription is up to date

> Make sure that levels of lighting are acceptable. Bright and poor lighting make it difficult for people to see each other

How to help overcome communication barriers caused by sight impairments

> Use alternative forms of communication that are chosen by the person, e.g. signing through touch and Braille

> Listen actively, using body language and eye contact, even if the person can't see you. They will be able to sense whether you are listening or not

> Check that you and the person have understood each other by asking questions and repeating the message

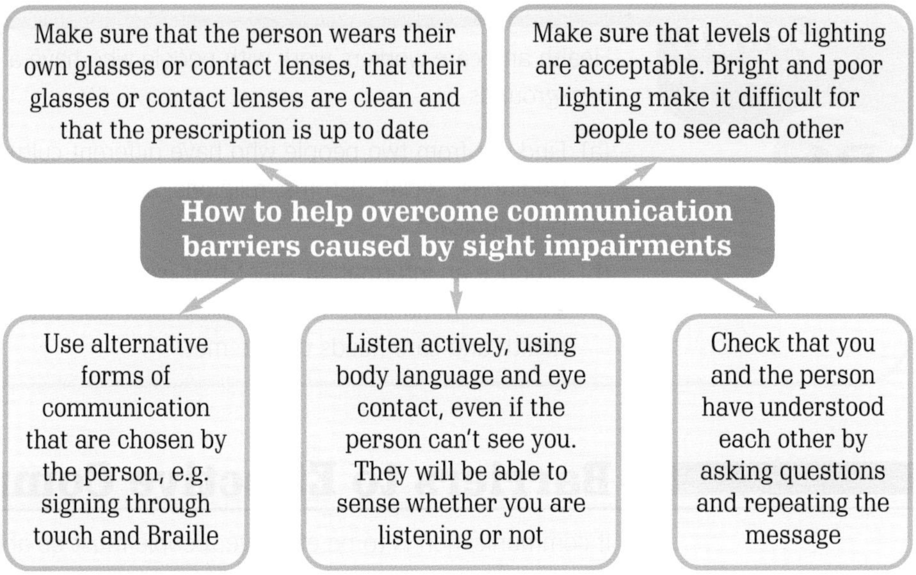

Language differences

Language differences can cause communication problems, for example:

- People from different countries speak different languages. If someone comes from a different country, try to learn their language or get help from a translator.

- People from different parts of the same country have different dialects, i.e. they have different accents and pronounce words differently. If you have an accent, speak slowly and clearly and check that you have been understood. If other people have an accent, check that you have understood them correctly.

- Workplace languages differ. People use different jargon (technical language) and acronyms (words formed by the initial letters of other words, e.g. Aids, NATO, RAM, etc.). Never use jargon or acronyms unless it is appropriate and you are confident that what you say will be understood. If other people use workplace language that you don't understand, always ask them to explain what they mean.

- People from different groups have their own slang words and expressions (very informal language). Never use slang if it would cause offence. If other people use slang that you don't understand, always ask them to explain what they mean.

Cultural differences

Cultural differences can cause communication problems. You have already looked at how communication differs between cultures. Because many of us don't know about or understand these differences, communication problems often exist between people from different cultures.

Health and care workers work with service users from a variety of cultural backgrounds. In order to meet their wants and needs, workers must understand cultural differences and know how to prevent any problems that might be caused by differences in communication.

Emotional issues

People's emotional state can cause communication barriers. For example, it can be difficult to communicate with people who are aggressive or who behave inappropriately (in ways that are unacceptable and which offend and upset others).

Figure 1.9

Communicating with people who are aggressive or have inappropriate behaviour

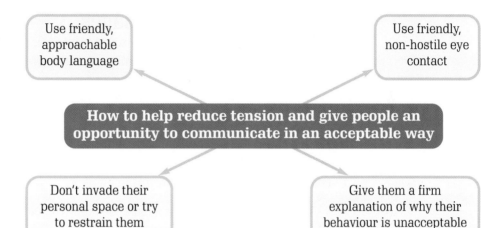

Use friendly, approachable body language

Use friendly, non-hostile eye contact

How to help reduce tension and give people an opportunity to communicate in an acceptable way

Don't invade their personal space or try to restrain them

Give them a firm explanation of why their behaviour is unacceptable

It can also be difficult to communicate with people who feel lonely and isolated or who are distressed because, for example, they have a life-threatening illness or a mental health condition such as dementia. Barriers caused by emotional issues like these can be overcome by:

- showing people that you understand their situation

- providing them with a safe and private environment in which to express themselves

- not rushing them. Giving people time to think through what they want to say and express themselves is very important.

Health problems and disabilities

These are also barriers to communication.

- A lack of mobility limits communication because it prevents people getting out and about and meeting up with others.

- Conditions brought on by a stroke make it difficult for people to speak and make themselves understood.

- Facial deformities and scars can make it difficult for people to use facial expressions to show their feelings.

- Conditions like cerebral palsy and Parkinson's disease make it difficult for people to control their muscles and use body language to express themselves.

Health and care workers can help reduce communication barriers caused by disabilities by understanding people's language needs, being patient and using active listening. Mobility equipment, such as wheelchairs and walking frames, helps people to socialise, but is only useful in adapted environments where there are wide doorways, ramps, lifts, etc.

Misinterpreting messages

Sometimes communication barriers exist because people misunderstand or misinterpret messages. It's easy to misinterpret a letter, telephone call, text message or email, because these types of communication don't contain any body language. We need to see people's body language to understand fully what they are telling us.

But even when body language is used, it can be easy to misinterpret a message, especially when someone is confused or has a learning difficulty. To help people understand what you tell them:

1. Repeat the message using expressions they can easily understand.
2. Give them sufficient time to absorb the information and try to understand it.
3. Ask them to repeat the message back to you, to confirm their understanding of the information it contained.

Figure 1.10
Not funny…

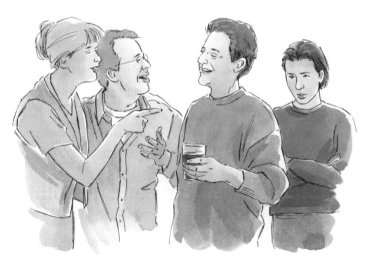

Jokes and humour are also easily misinterpreted. People don't laugh at the same things and can easily feel hurt or insulted by humour that they don't understand or don't like. Health and care workers should only use humour where they are confident that it is appropriate and that it will be understood.

Overcoming communication barriers

Here is a checklist for overcoming communication barriers.

1. Make sure the environment is quiet, well lit, warm, comfortable, safe and, if necessary, adapted for people with disabilities.

2. Know and understand how people need to communicate and use a form of communication that they choose.

3. If appropriate, use technological communication aids or human aids such as advocates, interpreters, translators and signers.

4. Speak clearly, use appropriate body language and listen actively to show you are interested and trying to understand what you are being told.

5. Check that you both understand each other correctly.

> **remember**
>
> Overcoming communication barriers is key to developing and maintaining good working relationships and meeting the needs of service users.

activity
INDIVIDUAL WORK
(1.4)

P2

Think about the different people you might meet as a care worker and make a list of barriers that could prevent you communicating effectively with them. Now suggest how these barriers could be overcome.

case study
1.1

Communication barriers at the Elms

The Elms is a residential care home for elderly people in the heart of a multicultural city. Many of the residents have dementia, are lonely, confused and depressed, and some have challenging behaviour. Most have mobility problems and sensory impairments. Residents and staff come from different parts of the world and have a variety of cultural backgrounds. Visiting health professionals use jargon when speaking to service users and acronyms when writing letters and making entries in care plans.

activity
GROUP WORK

(a) What communication barriers might exist at the Elms?

(b) Describe how these communication barriers might be overcome.

Diversity and Equality in Society

Diversity is to do with difference. We live in a society that is populated by people who are different because of their ethnicity, cultural background, gender, sexuality, family structure, social class and where they live and work.

Equality is to do with the fact that we are all as important as one another, despite our differences. It is about treating everyone fairly by giving them equal access to the same opportunities in life. Inequality is to do with treating people unfairly and in ways that don't value or respect them. When people are treated unfairly, they become victims of discrimination.

i Equal Opportunities Commission www.eoc.org.uk

In this section, you will learn about the factors that make us all different and the ways in which people are protected from unfair treatment.

The social factors that contribute to diversity

Social factors are the characteristics that are shared by a group of people. Our society is made up of a rich mix of different groups of people, each of which has its own individual characteristics.

Ethnicity

Ethnicity is to do with the cultural or national groups that people belong to. Different ethnic groups have their own distinctive characteristics, for example country of birth, skin colour and cultural background.

The 2001 Population Census categorised ethnic groups in the UK as follows:

Table 1.1 Population census

Ethnic group	People within the group
White	British, Irish, other White
Mixed	White and Black Caribbean, White and Black African, White and Asian, other mixed background
Asian or Asian British	Indian, Pakistani, Bangladeshi, other Asian background
Black or Black British	Caribbean, African, other Black background
Chinese or other ethnic group	Chinese, other ethnic group

Links to Unit 4, page 78.

Culture

Cultural backgrounds are different because of:

- the way people conduct their family lives and educate their children
- the attitudes, values and religious beliefs that people hold and pass down through the generations
- the traditions and customs that people respect and follow, e.g. ways of behaving, dressing, preparing and eating food.

People from different ethnic and cultural groups live, think and behave differently but are equally important and should have equal access to the same opportunities in life.

Gender and sexuality

Gender is to do with a person's sex. Broadly speaking, we fall into two groups – male and female. Different groups in society have different expectations of the way men and women should look and behave, and the society in which boys and girls grow up influences the roles they adopt as adults.

Despite their gender, men and women have different sexual preferences. Heterosexuals are attracted to people of the opposite sex, homosexuals (gay men and lesbians) are attracted to people of the same sex, and bisexuals are attracted to members of both sexes. These differences in sexuality contribute further to the diverse society in which we live.

Figure 1.11
Gender and age differences

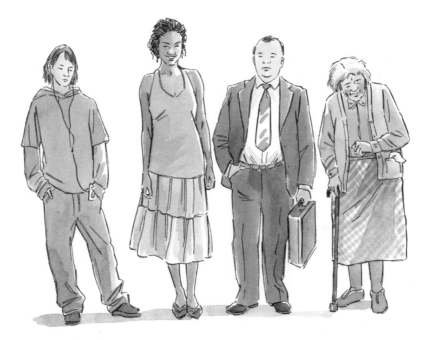

Men and women often think and behave differently but are equally important and should have equal access to the same opportunities in life.

Age

There are a number of different age groups in society. People are usually grouped as children, youths, young adults, middle-aged and elderly. People within each age group have shared experiences. They also have something different to offer society. For example, elderly people are wise and working adults make valuable contributions to the economy. In this way, each different age group contributes to the diversity in society.

People in different age groups may live, think and behave differently but are equally important and should have equal access to the same opportunities in life.

Family structure

Differences in family structure also contribute to a diverse society.

Table 1.2 Different family structures

Type of family	Family structure
Nuclear family	This is traditionally made up of a mother, father and their children, where the father is the 'breadwinner' and the woman looks after the home and the children. The nuclear family is often thought of as the 'normal' family group.
Extended family	This is made up of mother, father and the children, plus other relatives who either live close by or live with them in the same house. Extended families were more common in the past and are more common in less developed countries.
Single-parent family	This is usually the result of divorce or separation, or is where a parent has decided to bring his or her children up on their own. In the past, people often became single parents because of the death of their partner through childbirth, war or disease. These days, most single parents are mothers but statistics show that the number of single fathers is on the increase.
Reconstituted family	This is where people get married for a second, third, etc. time. Reconstituted families create step-parents and stepchildren.
Empty-nest family	This is where the children of a nuclear family have grown up and left home.
Single-person household	This is a household where the person lives on his or her own.
Same-sex parent family	This is where two women or two men live with their children, if they have any.

Whatever their structure, all families are equally important and should have equal access to the same opportunities in life.

Social class

Social class is another way of grouping people together. A person's social class is determined by their occupation, which is closely linked to their family background, education and geographical location (where they live). Because there are so many occupations in our society, there is a diverse range of social classes that people belong to, as the table below shows.

Table 1.3 The National Statistics Socio-economic Classifications (NS-SEC)

Level	Occupation
1	Higher managerial and professional occupations
1.1	Employers and managers in larger organisations, e.g. company directors, senior company managers, senior civil servants, senior officers in police and armed forces
1.2	Higher professionals, e.g. doctors, lawyers, clergy, teachers and social workers
2	Lower managerial and professional occupations, e.g. nurses and midwives, journalists, actors, musicians, prison officers, lower ranks of police and armed forces
3	Intermediate occupations, e.g. clerks, secretaries, driving instructors, telephone fitters
4	Small employers and own account workers, e.g. publicans, farmers, taxi drivers, window cleaners, painters and decorators
5	Lower supervisory, craft and related occupations, e.g. printers, plumbers, television engineers, train drivers, butchers
6	Semi-routine occupations, e.g. shop assistants, hairdressers, bus drivers, cooks
7	Routine occupations, e.g. couriers, labourers, waiters and refuse collectors
8	Those who have never had paid work and the long-term unemployed

Links to Unit 4, page 78.

Regardless of their social class, everyone is as important as each other and should have equal access to the same opportunities in life.

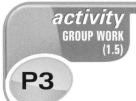

activity
GROUP WORK
(1.5)

P3

Look around your school, college or workplace and the neighbourhood in which you live. Make a list of the factors that contribute to the diversity and equality of the people that study, work and live there.

keyword

Service providers
Organisations that meet the needs of the public.

Policy
An official document that describes how an organisation aims to carry out its business.

Procedure
A way of doing things.

The political factors that protect diversity and equality

To protect people against unfair treatment and discrimination, governments produce legislation (laws, regulations and guidelines), and **service providers** and employers write **policies** and **procedures**. Legislation, policies and procedures are the political factors that protect the diversity and equality of workers, service users and the public.

You now know that equality is about treating everyone fairly by giving them the same opportunities in life. Inequality is to do with treating people unfairly and in ways that don't value or respect them.

Figure 1.12

Reasons why people may be treated unfairly

Their skin is the 'wrong' colour, e.g. white patients with mental health problems may be treated better than non-white patients with the same problems

They are the 'wrong' sex, e.g. women are less likely than men to be in higher paid jobs; and men are less likely to get jobs that women have traditionally worked in

Reasons why people may be treated unfairly

They are the 'wrong' age, e.g. younger people are more likely to be asked for their opinion than older people; and younger people are often unfairly accused of being yobs

They are disabled, e.g. people with physical disabilities find it very hard to access buildings and use public transport; and people with learning difficulties may not be welcomed within a community

The following laws ensure that we are all treated fairly and protected against discrimination. You will read more about discrimination in the next section.

- The Sex Discrimination Act 1975 states that men and women must be treated the same and have equal access to opportunities in life.

- The Disability Discrimination Act 1995 states that people who find it difficult to carry out day-to-day activities because of a disability should have the same opportunities in life as able-bodied people.

- The Race Relations Act 1976 states that everybody must be treated equally, regardless of their race, nationality or place of birth.

- The Equal Pay Act 1970 states that everyone has the right to the same pay and benefits where they are doing the same type of work.

- The Human Rights Act 1998 gives us general protection from discrimination.

Legislation banning unfair treatment on the grounds of age at work and in training is planned to come into force in 2006.

Service providers and employers obey these laws by writing anti-discriminatory policies and procedures, which describe how service users and the public are protected against unfair treatment. Health and social care workers have a responsibility to know their workplace policies and procedures. They can be held responsible for things that go wrong if they don't follow procedures.

The welfare state provides help and social support for people whose diverse needs prevent them accessing equal opportunities. For example, it provides them with a range of social security benefits, aims to improve their living conditions, promotes **community cohesion** and helps them into work. However, there are people whom, for one reason or another, the welfare state is not able to help. Private and voluntary organisations, and **informal carers**, play an important role in making sure these people are supported and treated fairly.

In 2000 the Government published the NHS Plan. This spells out how the National Health Service aims to meet the health needs of a diverse population in ways that are fair and do not discriminate. For example, the Plan states that the NHS:

- will provide a service for everyone that is based on need, not ability to pay

- will shape its services around the needs and preferences of individual patients, their families and their carers

- will respond to the needs of different groups and individuals within society, and challenge discrimination on the grounds of age, gender, ethnicity, religion, disability and sexuality

- will respond to different needs of different populations.

keyword

Community cohesion
Development of good relationships and equal opportunities between people from different backgrounds at work and in schools and neighbourhoods.

keyword

Informal carer
An unpaid carer, usually a friend or family member.

The National Health Service www.nhs.uk

Equality and non-discriminatory practice

Equality is about treating people fairly. Non-discriminatory work practice is a way of working that ensures people are treated fairly. This section aims to improve your understanding of what makes for discrimination and why non-discriminatory work practice is important.

Stereotyping and labelling

There are many different groups of people in society. We group people according to the one or two characteristics that they share, such as how they look and how they behave. Stereotyping happens when we assume that everyone in a group is the same in every way, for example that all elderly people or all disabled people are the same. Assuming that everyone in a group is the same in every way is too much of a generalisation and nearly always untrue.

A 'label' is a word we use to describe someone. Labels are usually based on people's appearance or behaviour. But labels can be offensive, for example 'wrinklies', 'Pakis' and 'benefits scroungers'. Another problem with labelling is that, instead of seeing a person as an individual, we only see their label. 'The hip replacement in bed number three' doesn't tell us much about the patient, only why they are in hospital and what bed they occupy!

Because stereotyping and labelling cause us to lose sight of the fact that everybody is unique, they are unfair ways of treating people. We might share one or two characteristics with other people but we all have different wants, needs, preferences, life experiences, expectations and family, cultural and ethnic backgrounds.

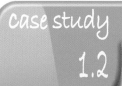

case study 1.2 — Stereotyping and labelling

A charitable organisation has applied for planning permission to build a community centre that caters for teenagers, families experiencing problems, elderly people, people with disabilities, learning difficulties and mental health problems, and people from ethnic minorities. A number of people in the neighbourhood have objected to the proposal and their local newspaper has accused them of discrimination.

activity
GROUP WORK

(a) What stereotypes do you think the objectors might hold for each of these groups of people?

(b) How do you think the objectors might have labelled the people who belong to the groups?

(c) Why is it not fair to stereotype or label these people?

(d) What effect might stereotyping and labelling have on them?

Prejudice and discrimination

'Prejudice' means to 'judge first', i.e. to make a judgement without any knowledge of what we are judging. A prejudice is a feeling or belief based on the way we prejudge someone. If we are positively prejudiced toward a person, we think well of them and what they do. If we are negatively prejudiced against a person, it's usually because they are different from us. We think less well of them than of people who are like us. Because prejudices are not based on facts, they are unfair.

Figure 1.13
Negative prejudices

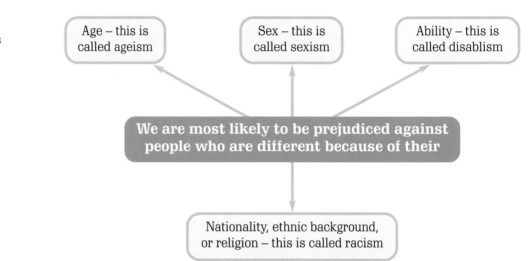

Discrimination happens when people let their prejudices and the way they stereotype and label people affect the way they treat others. Discrimination can be:

- ageist, for example when older people are forced to retire because they are considered to be 'past it' at work
- sexist, for example when women don't get promoted because employers think men are better at the job
- racist, for example when rioting occurs between different ethnic groups because each group thinks it is superior to the other
- disablist, for example when disabled people can't use services because their disability stops them accessing transport, buildings and information.

Discriminatory work practice happens when people let their prejudices and the way they stereotype and label people affect the way they work with others. People who practise discrimination at work are bullies. They harass and intimidate people, single them out and exclude them. As a result, their victims feel angry, unjustly treated, stressed and **oppressed**. They lose their self-confidence and self-worth, become demoralised and begin to feel unimportant, 'just a number'.

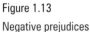

keyword

Oppression
Harsh, cruel treatment.

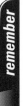

> **remember**
>
> Respecting and promoting diversity and equality is key to developing good working relationships and meeting the needs of service users.

Discriminatory work practice is against the law. As you read earlier, health and care workers have a responsibility to follow non-discriminatory work procedures. They must not let their prejudices and the way they label and stereotype others affect their work.

Discrimination stops people finding work and using services, which leads to poor living standards, poor health and family breakdown. People living like this are described as being 'deprived', and children growing up in deprivation do poorly at school. This means they will find it hard to gain employment. In the long term, discrimination results in cycles of deprivation for whole groups in society.

link

Links to Unit 4, pages 92–5.

> **activity**
> GROUP WORK
> (1.6)
>
> **M2**

Describe how the following factors might affect people's life chances:

(a) being a woman

(b) being gay

(c) being old

(d) being disabled

(e) belonging to a different ethnic or cultural background

(f) growing up in a single-parent family

(g) belonging to a low social class.

How the Principles of the Care Value Base Can be Used to Promote the Rights of Individuals and Significant Others

Individual rights

We all have rights. The anti-discrimination laws you read about above protect our right to equal treatment and to not be discriminated against. In addition, the Human Rights Act 1998 spells out our rights to:

■ respect, for our family and private life

■ freedom of expression, thought, religion and opinion

■ safety and protection of our personal possessions and protection from torture, slavery, abuse and punishment without a trial

■ freedom, unless we are suspected or convicted of committing a crime.

Whenever authorities, such as local authorities, health and social care providers, the police and magistrates make decisions about us, they have a duty to take our legal (lawful) rights into account. This ensures that we are treated fairly, decently and justly.

It isn't just the authorities who are obliged to take people's rights into account. We all have a moral duty to support each other's rights to:

- **be respected**
- **be treated as individuals**. Being labelled and stereotyped denies us the right to be treated as individuals.
- **dignity**. If our dignity is taken away, we lose our pride and can feel cheapened and degraded.
- **privacy**. We all have a right to privacy, for example in our relationships, correspondence, financial affairs, personal space and matters of personal hygiene. Loss of privacy can be distressing and lead to a loss of trust.
- **protection from danger and harm**. There are a number of laws that protect us from danger and harm.
- **access information about ourselves**. The Data Protection Act 1998 protects personal, sensitive information that we are often asked to give. It also allows us to see information that is recorded about us. For this reason, it is vitally important that all information is accurately recorded.
- **use our preferred method of communication and language**. You've already looked at the different ways people communicate and at why we must be given a choice about how we communicate.

Figure 1.14
Protecting our rights

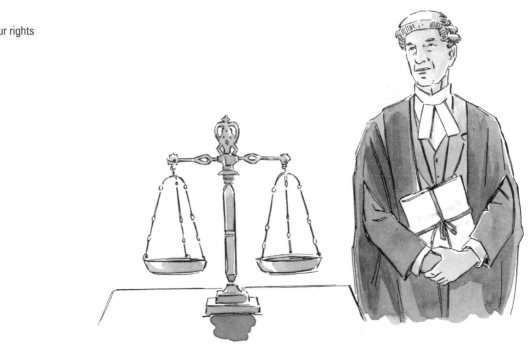

■ **be cared for in a way that meets our needs, takes account of our choices and protects us**. Our individual differences mean that we all have different health and care needs. We have a right to say how we want to be cared for and for that care to be delivered in ways that are safe.

Links to Unit 4, pages 97–100.

Links to Unit 4, pages 97–100.

activity
GROUP WORK
(1.7)

P4

Look at a charter of rights. Your workplace, school or college may have one. Alternatively, make a search on the Internet, where many organisations publish their charters. Using your research findings as a guide, draw up a 'Charter of Rights' that describes the rights of:

(a) your group at school or college or you and your colleagues at work

(b) users of health and social care services, e.g. people living in a residential care home.

The Care Value Base

The Care Value Base is a set of beliefs or values that shapes the way caring activities are carried out. By using the care values in their work, health and care workers can be confident that they support service users' rights to have:

■ Health and care workers who are caring, considerate and polite support service users' right to respect.

■ Health and care workers who recognise individual differences show service users that they are interested in the ways that people are different and how their differences affect their wants, needs, preferences and expectations. By responding to service users' differences in the way they work with them, they support service users' right to be treated as individuals.

■ Health and care workers who encourage service users to make choices help them stay in control of their lives and continue to feel good about themselves. They also support service users' rights to be cared for in ways that take account of their choices.

■ Health and care workers who respect service users' privacy show that they can be trusted and that they support their right to have a personal life and space and time to themselves. Common courtesy dictates that health and care workers knock before entering a room, wait to be asked to read someone else's mail, and move away when someone is on the phone.

■ Health and care workers who help service users stay independent and responsible for themselves show that they value them for what they can and can't do. They also show that they want them to continue to achieve and feel fulfilled. By encouraging independence in a safe and secure environment, health and care workers support service users' rights to be treated as individuals and protected from danger and harm.

- Health and care workers who recognise service users' dignity show that they appreciate their need for self-respect. They also show that they value service users' sense of what is correct, their way of doing things and their way of presenting themselves. Promoting pride and self-respect supports service users' rights to be treated with dignity.

- Health and care workers who work in partnership with service users show that they value their knowledge and experience. Working in partnership supports service users' rights to be treated as individuals, to be cared for in ways that meet their needs, to communicate in ways with which they are comfortable, and to be allowed access to information about themselves.

Health and care workers have a responsibility to use the Care Value Base in their work. The care values and how they must be used in work activities are described in job descriptions, workplace policies, procedures and **mission statements**, service users' care plans, and **charters** produced for service users by service providers.

Links to Unit 4, page 99.

Some workers have additional **codes of practice** and charters to work to.

Health care workers have to abide by the Patients' Charter, which covers patients' rights, the standards set by the Healthcare Commission and the NHS Knowledge and Skills Framework (NHS KSF).

Social care workers have to follow standards and codes of practice, including those set out by the Commission for Social Care Inspection, the General Social Care Council and the Sector Skills Council 'Skills for Care and Development'.

And because health and care workers work in partnership with service users, they must always be guided by the expectations of people receiving the service and their needs and preferences.

Healthcare Commission www.chai.org.uk
Commission for Social Care Inspection www.csci.org.uk
General Social Care Council www.gscc.org.uk
Sector Skills Councils 'Skills for Care and Development' www.skillsforcare.org.uk

Health and care workers' responsibilities

We all have rights but with rights come responsibilities. The most important responsibility for health and care workers is to uphold service users' rights.

You read earlier that to care appropriately, health and care workers need to be able to communicate with service users. For this reason, they also have a responsibility to support service users' rights to communicate their needs, views and preferences.

keyword

Mission statement
An organisation's mission statement describes what it is, what it does, its values and its beliefs.

Charter
A description of an organisation's purpose.

keyword

Code of practice
A set of rules.

Cultural and language differences, disabilities, sensory impairments and emotional issues can prevent communication. If health and care workers don't overcome communication barriers, service users' needs, views and preferences won't be made clear. As a result, they may not be cared for in ways that take account of their diversity, and they may be cared for inappropriately and less favourably than others. Denying people their right to fair treatment and equal opportunities is against the law.

Confidentiality

To care appropriately, health and care workers need to know a great deal of very personal information about service users. They have a responsibility to protect service users' right to privacy by keeping this information confidential. Confidentiality is about privacy and protecting personal information.

The Data Protection Act 1998 is in place to make sure that personal information is protected. Workplace confidentiality policies and procedures spell out exactly how everyone is required to deal with confidential information. As a rule of thumb, no one should be allowed access to anyone else's personal information unless they have:

■ been given permission by that person

■ a right or a need to know the information.

It is also very important that:

■ information is stored securely. Manual (paper) records and reports must be filed correctly in a locked filing cabinet or kept in a locked office, for which there is a named key holder. Electronic records must be stored in computer files that can only be opened by people who have a secure password.

■ workplace procedures for retrieving information from storage are followed, e.g. by getting permission from the key holder or a superior

Figure 1.15
Maintaining confidentiality

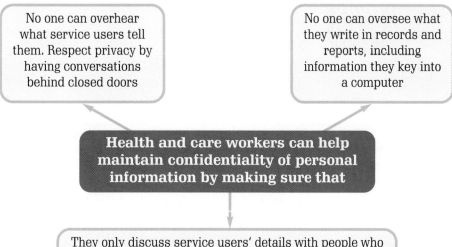

No one can overhear what service users tell them. Respect privacy by having conversations behind closed doors

No one can oversee what they write in records and reports, including information they key into a computer

Health and care workers can help maintain confidentiality of personal information by making sure that

They only discuss service users' details with people who have a right or a need to know, e.g. other health and care workers; and that discussions take place in private

- when records and reports have been taken out of storage, great care must be taken to make sure they are only seen by people who have a right or need to know their contents

- when records and reports are finished with, they are promptly returned to storage.

Disclosing information

There are occasions when confidentiality needs to be 'broken' and personal information passed on without a person's permission, for example if there are concerns about abuse. This is known as disclosure, and, unless there are exceptional circumstances, the person must be told without delay exactly what information has been disclosed.

Disclosing information about someone can be difficult because of the tension between rights and responsibilities. Health and care workers have a responsibility to protect service users' rights to privacy, and breaking confidentiality can seem to deny them this right. However, disclosure is never carried out without good reason.

Situations where there are tensions between rights and responsibilities include:

- rude, aggressive service users who upset and intimidate others. Whilst everyone has a right to express themselves, they also have a responsibility to protect other people's right to respect for their private life.

- elderly service users who live independently but who may be forgetful and forget to lock doors, turn appliances off, etc. Whilst people have a right to remain independent, they also have a responsibility to protect other people's right to safety and security.

Health and care workers have a responsibility to know how to deal with tensions between rights and responsibilities. Common sense, experience, and getting help from colleagues can help find a balance.

> **remember**
>
> Respecting and promoting individual rights is key to developing and maintaining good working relationships and meeting the needs of service users.

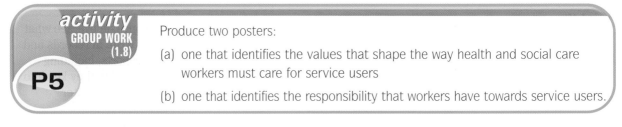

activity
GROUP WORK
(1.8)

P5

Produce two posters:

(a) one that identifies the values that shape the way health and social care workers must care for service users

(b) one that identifies the responsibility that workers have towards service users.

activity
INDIVIDUAL WORK
(1.9)

M3

D2

Visit your local GP practice, drop-in centre or a Social Services/private social care setting. Talk to staff to find out:

(a) how the care values and their responsibilities to service users promote service users' rights

(b) how they use the care values and carry out their responsibilities to promote service users' rights

progress check

1. Give five examples of communication skills that contribute to the success of one-to-one and group interactions.
2. Describe five examples of barriers to effective communication and how each can be overcome.
3. Give five examples of how a health or care worker can use communication skills to promote effective communication with service users.
4. Give six examples of factors that contribute to the diversity and equality of society.
5. Describe how people's equality can be affected by these factors.
6. Describe five examples of service users' rights.
7. What are the care values?
8. Explain how using the care values allows health and care workers to support and promote service users' rights.
9. Give five examples of care workers' responsibilities to service users.
10. Explain how health and care workers' responsibilities support and promote service users' rights.

Books

Blundell, J. (2001), *Active Sociology for GCSE* (Longman)

Burnard, P. and Morrison, P. (1997), *Caring and Communicating* (Palgrave Macmillan)

Meggitt, C. (1997), *A Special Needs Handbook for Health and Social Care* (Hodder Arnold)

Michie, V. (2004), *Working in Care Settings* (Nelson Thornes)

Miller, J. (1996), *Social Care Practice* (Hodder and Stoughton)

Nolan, Y. (2003), *S/NVQ Level 2 in Care: Student Handbook* (Heinemann)

Richards, A. (1999), *The Complete A–Z Health and Social Care Handbook* (Hodder Arnold)

Windsor, G. and Moonie, N. (ed) (2000) *GNVQ Health and Social Care: Intermediate Compulsory Units with Edexcel Options* (Heinemann)

Other publications

General Social Care Council (2002), *Codes of Practice for Social Care Workers and Employers*

Health and social care providers' policies, procedures and charters

The NHS Plan

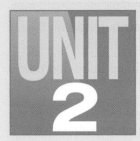

Individual Needs within the Health and Social Care Sectors

This unit covers:

- the needs of individuals in society
- factors that influence the health and needs of individuals
- hazards in health and social care environments
- health and safety legislation and guidelines.

We all have physical, emotional, social and intellectual needs. Understanding and meeting the needs of service users is key to good care practice. It is also important to understand the factors that influence people's health and needs and the hazards that affect their health and safety. Service users are more exposed to health and safety hazards because of their vulnerability. There are a number of laws that aim to protect their right to health and safety and these are written into workplace policies and procedures. Good care practice dictates that health and care workers follow health and safety procedures in their work with service users.

grading criteria

To achieve a **Pass** grade the evidence must show that the learner is able to:	To achieve a **Merit** grade the evidence must show that the learner is able to:	To achieve a **Distinction** grade the evidence must show that the learner is able to:
P1 describe the everyday needs of individuals in society Pg 32	**M1** explain the potential effects of four factors that can influence the health and subsequent needs of individuals in society. Pg 44	**D1** explain the potential physical, social and emotional effects on the individual achieving the targets in the action plan Pg 46
P2 identify the potential effects of four factors that can influence the health and subsequent needs of individuals in society Pg 44	**M2** describe factors which may influence the ability of an individual to adhere to an action plan Pg 46	**D2** explain the strengths and weaknesses of actions taken to minimise risks in health and social care environments Pg 52

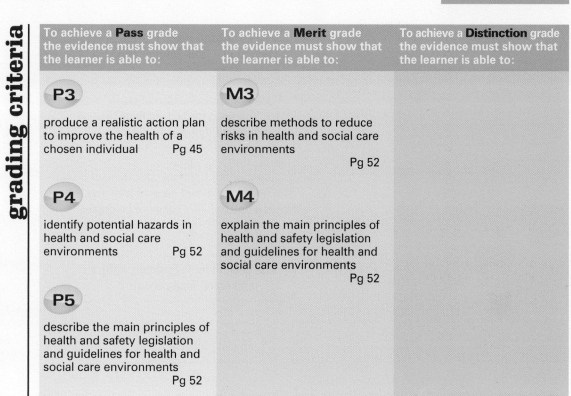

grading criteria

To achieve a **Pass** grade the evidence must show that the learner is able to:	To achieve a **Merit** grade the evidence must show that the learner is able to:	To achieve a **Distinction** grade the evidence must show that the learner is able to:
P3 produce a realistic action plan to improve the health of a chosen individual Pg 45	**M3** describe methods to reduce risks in health and social care environments Pg 52	
P4 identify potential hazards in health and social care environments Pg 52	**M4** explain the main principles of health and safety legislation and guidelines for health and social care environments Pg 52	
P5 describe the main principles of health and safety legislation and guidelines for health and social care environments Pg 52		

The Needs of Individuals in Society

We all have **needs**. To enjoy good health and a sense of well-being, our needs have to be met.

Maslow's hierarchy of needs

Abraham Maslow (1908–70) was a psychologist who suggested that our ability to reach our full potential and have a good quality of life depends on our needs being met in a certain order. He defined a **hierarchy** of needs.

Our basic physical needs, for example food, water, shelter and warmth, are the most important. People who are homeless, hungry and cold are more interested in finding a warm bed for the night and having a meal than in keeping themselves safe or making friends.

When our basic physical needs are met, we can take steps to meet our need for physical safety and emotional security, for instance by steering clear of situations and people that are unsafe or cause us anxiety.

When we feel safe and secure, we can develop relationships that meet our need to give and receive love and affection and in which we feel accepted and have a sense of belonging.

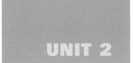

Figure 2.1
Maslow's hierarchy of needs

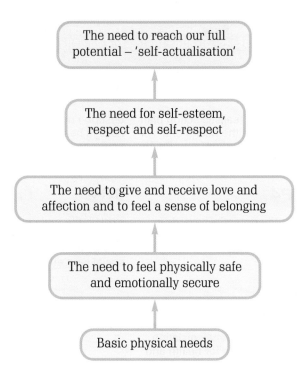

When we are able to form successful relationships we develop **self-confidence**, **self-esteem** and **self-respect**. In addition, other people respect us.

When we are self-confident and have self-esteem and self-respect, we can go on to achieve our full potential or, as Maslow said, to achieve 'self-actualisation'. People achieve self-actualisation through developing new skills and meeting new challenges. 'Self-actualisers' are satisfied with their lives. Unfortunately, most of us spend so much time worrying about meeting our basic needs, staying safe and secure and our relationships that we don't give ourselves a chance to reach our full potential!

keyword

Self-confidence
To be confident in your own abilities.

Self-esteem
To have a good opinion about yourself.

Self-respect
To feel you behave in an admirable and correct way.

keyword

Diet
The food we eat on a day-to-day basis.

keyword

Hazard
A source of danger

keyword

Hypothermia
abnormally low blood temperature.

Physical needs

We all have the same basic physical needs, which include:

- **water** and a nutritious and balanced **diet**, to stay healthy.
- **physical activity**, which keeps us healthy and prevents us putting on weight. This in turn helps us look and feel good about ourselves.
- **shelter**. People who are homeless or living in run-down, overcrowded conditions are exposed to health and safety **hazards** that affect their physical and mental health.
- **warmth**, to maintain our body temperature and stay comfortable. A drop in body temperature leads to **hypothermia**, which can be life threatening.
- **safety**. Living and working in hazardous situations and experiencing threats and intimidation can lead to physical and mental ill health.

Figure 2.2

Plenty of exercise, water and a balanced diet are key physical needs

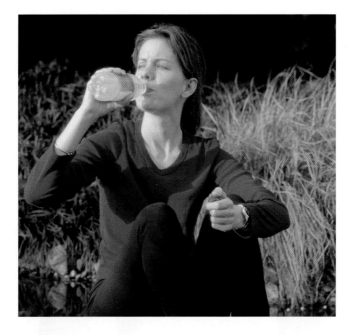

Social needs

We all need to be able to develop and maintain relationships with family, friends, the people we work with and the people in the groups we are members of. Relationships satisfy our need to belong. They protect us from isolation and loneliness and give us an opportunity to mix with different people, learn how to cooperate and develop new skills.

Most of us also have a need to be accepted by others. If we aren't accepted, we lose confidence and self-esteem. In order to be accepted, some people behave in ways that make them feel uncomfortable. Pretending to be someone we aren't makes life difficult and doesn't make for successful relationships.

Emotional needs

We all have a need to give and receive love and affection. We satisfy this need by developing emotional bonds or relationships with other people. Babies and children who are given lots of love and affection are able to develop loving, affectionate, supportive relationships with other people throughout their lives.

Receiving love and affection and being emotionally fulfilled helps us develop self-esteem and self-confidence. As Maslow said, when we have developed self-esteem, we are ready to go on to achieve our full potential.

Intellectual needs

Intellectual needs are to do with keeping our brains stimulated and active. We all have the same intellectual needs, which include being able to communicate with other people, to learn and understand, to think and solve problems, to remember, and to achieve and feel fulfilled.

Figure 2.3
Self-esteem breeds success

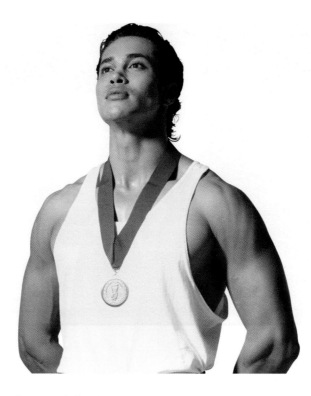

Everyone's intellectual needs can be met through stimulating environments. For example, children learn and develop communication skills through the stimulation offered in playgroups and schools; and an adult's need to achieve is met through the stimulation of challenging environments, for example, at work or in their career.

Achievement, like belonging and acceptance, leads to the development of self-esteem. And as you know, having self-esteem helps us to develop our full potential. This is why it is important that we continue to meet our intellectual needs all through our lives.

In addition to having basic needs, we each have specific needs, which depend on our individual circumstances. For example, someone with diabetes has specific dietary needs; someone who is disabled may need help to be physically active; and someone who is confused may need help remembering the day of the week. You will read more about specific needs shortly.

remember

We all have needs. Satisfying a person's needs is key to their health and well-being and helps them develop their potential.

activity
INDIVIDUAL WORK
(2.1)

P1

(a) Make a list of your physical, social, emotional and intellectual needs.

(b) Describe how each need is met.

(c) Why is it important that each of your needs is met?

Factors that Influence the Health and Needs of Individuals

Our health and needs are influenced by a number of different factors.

Physical factors that influence our health and needs

Biological inheritance

One of the reasons we are all different is that we each have a unique set of **genes** (apart from identical **siblings**, who have the same set of genes as each other). We inherit our genes from our parents, which is why we resemble them.

Genes can become defective and cause genetic diseases such as cystic fibrosis, Huntington's disease and haemophilia.

Cystic fibrosis is a genetic disease that affects a number of organs in the body by clogging them up with thick, sticky mucus. People with cystic fibrosis have special care needs, which include:

- physiotherapy to help drain mucus away from their lungs
- special medication to treat the parts of the body that are affected by the disease
- a healthy diet to fight chest infections.

The Cystic Fibrosis Trust www.cftrust.org.uk

Huntington's disease causes uncontrollable body movements, depression and a loss of social and intellectual skills. In addition to having basic needs, people with Huntington's chorea have special care needs, which include:

- help to move, communicate and eat
- help with understanding other people's needs and emotions
- help remembering.

The Huntington's Disease Association www.hda.org.uk

Haemophilia is a disease in which the blood doesn't clot properly so that sufferers bleed for longer than normal. In addition to having basic needs, people with haemophilia have special care needs, which include:

- protection in situations that can cause bleeding, e.g. minor surgery, dental surgery
- the need for blood products that help prevent or control bleeding.

The Haemophilia Society www.haemophilia.org.uk

Genes are carried on chromosomes. The normal number of chromosomes in human beings is 46 but sometimes a baby is born with too many or too few. Conditions caused by the wrong number of chromosomes are called chromosome disorders.

An example of a chromosome disorder is Down's syndrome. People with Down's syndrome have special care needs because:

- their physical and intellectual development is slow
- their eyesight may be poor
- they may have congenital heart disease
- they may suffer from chest and ear infections, which can lead to deafness
- they may have poor muscle tone. Babies with Down's syndrome are often quite floppy.

The Down's Syndrome Association www.downs-syndrome.org.uk

Environment

Another important physical influence on our health and needs is the **environment** in which we live.

keyword

Environment
The physical surroundings and conditions that affect our lives.

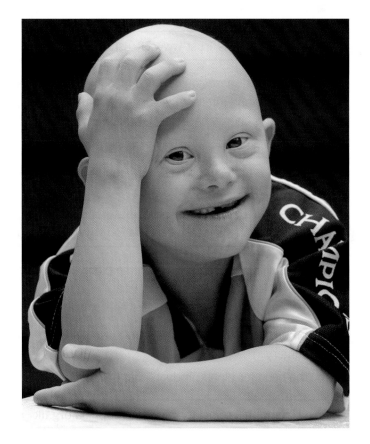

Figure 2.4

Child with Down's syndrome

The environment in which a baby lives whilst in the uterus (womb) affects their growth and development. For example, if a pregnant woman:

- catches German measles, her baby may suffer brain damage
- smokes, her baby may be small, weak and suffer with lung infections
- drinks alcohol, her baby may be born with foetal alcohol syndrome (brain damage and deformity of the face)
- doesn't eat a well-balanced diet that includes folic acid, her baby may develop spina bifida (a defect of the spinal cord).

The environment into which we are born also has countless effects on our health and needs. For example, the air we breathe is polluted by airborne **micro-organisms**, dust, pollen, smoke, exhaust fumes and chemicals used at home and at work. Air pollution causes:

- breathing problems, e.g. asthma
- acute respiratory infections, e.g. bronchitis
- chronic, lifelong respiratory diseases, e.g. asbestosis and emphysema.

People with respiratory problems are treated with inhalers, oxygen, antibiotics and drugs.

The quality of the water we drink and use for preparing food influences our health. For example, water polluted by poisonous bacteria can cause diarrhoea and cholera; and water polluted by chemicals can slow down a child's development and cause cancer. Bottled water is a safe alternative to polluted tap water; and good personal hygiene helps prevent the spread of infections caused by waterborne bacteria.

Noise is a form of pollution. We are exposed to noise at home, school, college and work; from neighbours, traffic and animals; and in shops and at events. Noise can be stressful; it makes communication difficult; it disturbs our sleep and damages our ears, resulting in deafness. People whose hearing is impaired can be helped by hearing aids and sign language.

We all benefit from small amounts of the sun's ultraviolet (UV) radiation but overexposure causes skin cancer and cataracts. Skin cancer can be fatal if not caught in time. Cataracts cloud the lens in the eye, causing sight impairments. Treatment is by removing the clouded lens and replacing it with an artificial one.

Where we live has an impact on our health and needs. Some areas of the world are more likely than others to experience environmental disasters such as volcanic activity, **tsunamis** and earthquakes. Others are more exposed to extreme weather conditions, such as floods, hurricanes and droughts. The effects of environmental disasters and extreme weather on health and needs include malnutrition, starvation, dehydration, hypothermia, infectious disease, physical injury, mental ill health and death.

keyword

Micro-organisms
Minute organisms, e.g. bacteria, which can only be seen through a microscope lens.

keyword

Tsunami
A long, high sea wave caused by an underwater earthquake.

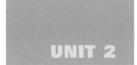

Figure 2.5

Environmental disasters can affect our health and needs

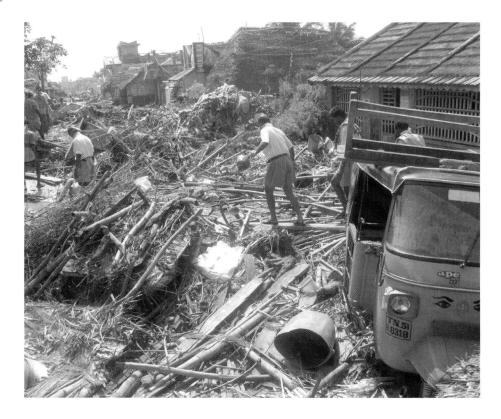

Socio-economic factors that influence our health and needs

Social class and income

Social class and income affect our health and well-being. The higher our social class, the more money we have to spend. Being financially comfortable means that we can, if we choose, spend more money on basic health needs, such as nutritious food, housing and heating. It means we can choose to join a gym, take relaxing and stimulating holidays, have an active social life and indulge ourselves. As a result, we experience good health and well-being.

On the other hand, the lower our social class, the less money we have to spend. As a consequence, our basic needs may not be adequately met and our health and well-being suffer.

Employment

Employment affects our health and well-being in many ways. It allows us to earn money to spend on our basic health needs. It can also stimulate our minds and give us an opportunity to build relationships. Employment meets our need to belong and helps build our self-confidence and self-esteem. Being in employment helps us maintain a good quality of life and keeps us healthy.

Unemployment can lead to poverty and physical ill health. It can also lead to mental ill health because of loneliness and social isolation.

Housing

Housing is a basic health need. We all have a right to decent, affordable housing that provides warmth and protection. Homelessness and cold, damp, overcrowded, insecure and filthy living conditions cause physical ill health, breakdown in relationships and emotional and social isolation.

Education

Education is important for health and well-being. Knowledge and skills go hand in hand with being employed and earning enough money to buy basic health necessities and have a good quality of life. Education also encourages us to think about our lifestyle and to make choices that promote our health and well-being.

Figure 2.6

The influence of income, employment, housing and education on health and needs

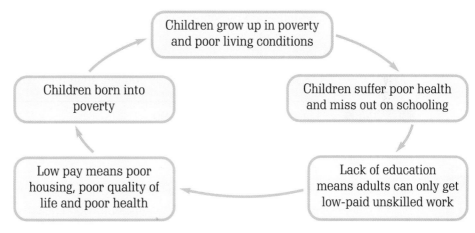

Accessibility of services

To stay in good health, we have to be able to access (use) health and care services when we need them, including services that provide education, social security benefits and help with employment and housing.

People can experience problems accessing services if, for example:

- they don't know that the service exists
- they don't know how to access the service
- they are old and frail, have a communication difficulty, are physically disabled or have a mental health problem or learning difficulty
- the service provider is not represented in the area where they live
- transport to and from the service provider is difficult for them to use, is expensive or is infrequent.

Gender

Gender influences health and needs because men and women have variations in body structure and function and often think and behave differently. For example, women have a higher rate of **morbidity** but men have a higher rate of early **mortality**, in particular from coronary heart disease. Women are more likely to use health screening services than men, possibly because they are the family carer and need to stay well. Men are more likely than women to commit suicide and to have accidents at work, whilst women have more accidents in the home.

keyword

Morbidity
Illness.

Mortality
Death.

37

Culture and religion

Cultural differences between people are based on their traditions, social customs, religion and personal preferences. These differences influence people's health and needs, for example:

■ Dietary needs: practising Muslims are only allowed to eat halal meat, and vegetarians choose not to eat meat.

■ Medication needs: Jehovah's Witnesses choose not to have blood transfusions, and people who don't eat meat won't take medication that contains animal products.

■ Physical care needs: people from some cultures are uncomfortable being seen undressed by someone of the opposite sex, and Orthodox Jewish women must not be touched whilst they are having a period.

■ Courtesy needs: some people prefer to be addressed formally, e.g. Mrs Smith, especially by people younger than themselves.

link

Links to Unit 4, pages 81–90.

The media

keyword

Signs
The visible marks of an illness, e.g. swollen glands.

Symptoms
The feelings that accompany an illness, e.g. a headache.

The media, e.g. TV, radio, film, newspapers and magazines, have an influence on our health and needs by running campaigns that promote, for example, healthy eating, safe sex and giving up smoking. Good health is also promoted by the media in advertisements, sitcoms and soaps, plays, documentaries, interviews with health professionals and service users, and so on.

In addition, the media educate us about the **signs** and **symptoms** of health conditions, and about new procedures and technologies that have been developed to meet our health and care needs.

Lifestyle factors that influence our health and needs

Our lifestyle is to do with the way we choose to live. The choices we make affect our health and needs.

keyword

Anus
The opening in a person's bottom through which faeces (waste material) is excreted from the body.

Genitals
Sexual organs.

Personal hygiene

Good personal hygiene is closely linked to good health. Personal hygiene is about:

■ keeping our body clean, especially areas that sweat and can smell, such as feet, armpits, **anus** and **genitals**

■ keeping our clothes clean and tidy

■ washing our hands after using the toilet and before and after working with food.

A good standard of personal hygiene helps prevent the spread of infection between people and to and from food. It also ensures that we look presentable. People who look presentable earn respect and as a result develop self-respect and self-confidence.

Figure 2.7
Nice to work with

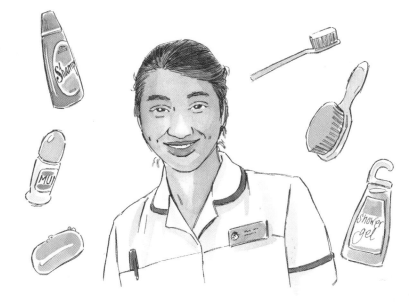

Many activities in health and care settings involve being physically close to service users. For this reason, health and care workers need to have very high standards of personal hygiene.

Diet

Our diet influences our health and needs in many ways. You read earlier that we need water and a balanced diet to stay healthy. If we don't get the balance right we:

■ gain weight and become obese, which increases our risk of getting heart disease and breathing problems

■ lose weight, which increases our risk of catching infections

■ suffer from 'nutritional deficiency' conditions such as anaemia and brittle bone disease.

Obesity and weight loss can also affect our self-esteem, because we lose pride in our appearance. This in turn can lead to social isolation.

Everybody's dietary needs are different and are described in Unit 9.

Links to Unit 9, page 201.

Health and care workers play a very important role in the lives of service users, and their work activities require them to be healthy and to have a great deal of energy. For these reasons, it is essential that they eat a nutritious, well-balanced diet that controls their weight.

Physical exercise

The amount of physical exercise we have affects our health and needs. Increasing the amount of exercise we do doesn't have to mean going to the gym every day! It can be as simple and easy as:

- walking to school, college or work instead of driving or catching the bus
- using the stairs instead of the lift
- washing the car yourself instead of taking it to the car wash.

Figure 2.8

The benefits of exercise

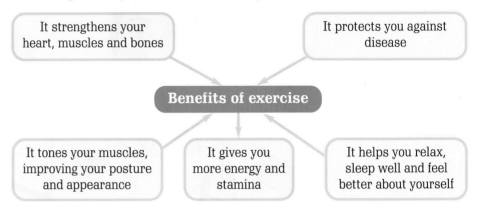

It strengthens your heart, muscles and bones

It protects you against disease

Benefits of exercise

It tones your muscles, improving your posture and appearance

It gives you more energy and stamina

It helps you relax, sleep well and feel better about yourself

Health and care workers not only need to eat well, they need to take plenty of physical exercise so that they have enough strength, energy and stamina to do their job.

Stress

Stress plays a part in everybody's lives. A little stress can be stimulating but too much can damage our health. The emotional effects of stress include not being able to cope, frustration, anger and depression. The physical effects include headaches, tense muscles, sleep problems, asthma, ulcers, cold sores, coughs, colds and high blood pressure.

There are many different ways of coping with stress. For example, you could do something that uses up the excess energy that stress produces; you could talk your feelings through with someone who is prepared to listen; and you could use relaxation techniques, such as breathing exercises, when you feel the need. Health and care workers meet stressful situations on a daily basis. They need to be able to deal with stress before it affects their health.

Sexual practice

For people who are in secure, loving, adult relationships, sex is a meaningful way of giving and receiving love. However, some sexual practices are physically and emotionally dangerous. For example, **unprotected sex** can result in unplanned pregnancies and the spread of sexually transmitted infections (STIs).

keyword

Unprotected sex Having sex without using any contraception, which may lead to pregnancy or catching a sexually transmitted infection.

The Teenage Pregnancy Unit www.teenagepregnancyunit.gov.uk
National Health Service Direct www.nhsdirect.nhs.uk

Unplanned pregnancies are avoided by using contraceptives. Contraceptives include the condom, the diaphragm, the pill, the coil (intrauterine device – IUD) and the rhythm (natural) method. Sterilisation is also an option for some people.

Sexually transmitted infections usually cause itching, swelling or redness around the vagina or penis, an unusual discharge from the vagina or penis, or pains in the lower abdomen. STIs include chlamydia, gonorrhoea, genital herpes, pubic lice, scabies, HIV, syphilis and thrush.

You can never be 100 per cent sure that a sexual partner doesn't have an STI, and the more sexual partners you have, the higher the risk of catching one. The most effective way to prevent STIs is to use the male condom.

Substance abuse

Substance abuse can have disastrous effects on health. For example, excessive use of alcohol can cause:

- heart disease, high blood pressure, stroke and cirrhosis of the liver
- personality changes, which affect work and social relationships
- increased **reaction time**, which results in accidents
- depression and suicide.

> **keyword**
>
> **Reaction time**
> The time it takes for someone to respond to a stimulus or change in the situation.

Table 2.1 The classification of illegal drugs

Classification	Examples of drugs
Class A	These are the most dangerous drugs and include cocaine, heroin, opium and ecstasy.
Class B	These are dangerous but less so than class A drugs. They include amphetamines and barbiturates.
Class C	These are also harmful but the least harmful of the three classes. They include cannabis and Valium.

Legal drugs are drugs that a doctor can prescribe or which we can buy over the counter. Illegal drugs are drugs that are banned by the law. Doctors can prescribe some of them for relieving medical symptoms but they're not legal in any other circumstances.

Drug abuse means using illegal, prescription-only and over-the-counter drugs for reasons for which they are not intended. Because illegal drugs often contain substances that are much more harmful than the drugs themselves, using them is extremely risky to health. Both illegal and legal drugs can be addictive, and heavy or long-term use can cause overdose and death.

Solvent abuse involves inhaling substances called solvents, such as butane and propane. Solvents are found in gas refills and lighters and in some aerosols, air fresheners, paint thinners, correcting fluids and glues. Solvents are sniffed for their intoxicating effects. However, the risks to health, which can be fatal, far outweigh the intoxicating effects of the gases.

www.bbc.co.uk/crime/drugs

may feel that they are being discriminated against. They become disheartened, lose self-confidence and self-esteem and can become aggressive. In the long term, they find it difficult to show their feelings and difficult to build relationships. They lose their sense of belonging and become withdrawn, lonely and isolated.

Sexual abuse

Sexual abuse happens when people are sexually harassed, exposed to unwelcome sexual activity, for example touched inappropriately, or used to sexually gratify the abuser. People who were sexually abused as children may grow up to be abusers themselves.

The signs of sexual abuse include bleeding, bruising, swelling, STIs and unwanted pregnancies. In the short term, victims of sexual abuse can feel disgusted, humiliated, embarrassed and frightened. In the medium term, they may feel ashamed, degraded and lose their dignity and self-respect. In the long term, they may become withdrawn and unable to develop loving sexual relationships.

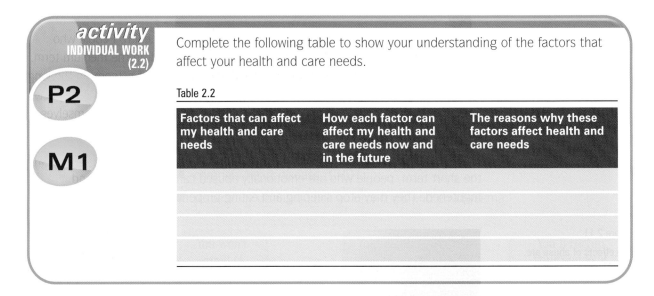

activity
INDIVIDUAL WORK
(2.2)

P2

M1

Complete the following table to show your understanding of the factors that affect your health and care needs.

Table 2.2

Factors that can affect my health and care needs	How each factor can affect my health and care needs now and in the future	The reasons why these factors affect health and care needs

case study   **Stephen**

2.1

Stephen, aged 14, has been knocked about by his father for as long as he can remember. His father also teases him about his physical appearance.

activity
GROUP WORK

(a) In what ways is Stephen being abused by his father?

(b) How might his father's behaviour affect Stephen's health and needs now and in the future?

Planning for good health

In the last few pages, you've read about a range of factors that influence our health and needs. Has reading about them prompted you to make any changes? You might have tried to improve your health in the past, for example by stopping smoking or losing weight. How successful we are at health-improvement changes depends on the goals we set ourselves.

It's a smart idea to set SMART goals (objectives) when planning to improve health. SMART goals are:

- **S**pecific : clear and precise
- **M**easurable : so we can find out whether we have been successful
- **A**chievable : possible and within reach
- **R**ealistic : sensible and practical
- **T**ime-related : because it helps to have a deadline to work to.

Think about these two health improvement goals:

1. 'I want to lose a stone over the next three months.'
2. 'I want to lose loads of weight as soon as possible.'

The first goal is very specific. It talks about losing a specific amount of weight over a specific period of time. The second goal is not clear. What precisely do 'loads of weight' and 'as soon as possible' mean?

The first goal is measurable. Although you can get on the scales to see if you've lost weight, 'loads' isn't a measurement. It's much more helpful to check for a measurable amount of weight loss.

The first goal is achievable. Weight-loss programmes recommend a weight loss rate of one and a half to two pounds a week. Losing one and a half pounds a week over three months is a weight loss of about 18 pounds, which is more than a stone. Starving ourselves or going on a crash diet would be the only way to lose 'loads of weight as soon as possible'. However, giving up eating or sticking to a crash diet is easier said than done! So the second goal is not achievable.

The first goal is realistic or sensible. Losing weight slowly by making sensible changes to what we eat and the amount of exercise we take will help ensure that the weight stays off. The second goal is not sensible because losing 'loads of weight' in a very short space of time is not healthy. It's also not sensible because weight that is lost quickly goes back on again just as quickly!

Unlike the second goal, the first goal is time-related. It has a deadline. All plans benefit from having deadlines. If you don't have deadlines or you only have a vague deadline, such as 'as soon as possible', you can't keep a check on your progress.

activity
INDIVIDUAL WORK
(2.3)

P3

Identify two or three health improvement goals that you would like to achieve and write yourself a SMART action plan that will help you to achieve each goal.

remember
A multitude of factors influences our health and needs. Some we can't control but others we can, by maintaining a healthy lifestyle.

If we don't achieve our goals, we need to ask ourselves why. Did we give ourselves enough time? Or did social and financial factors prevent us losing weight? For example, we may not have much choice about the meals that are prepared for us; going for a run every day can be lonely and extremely boring, and menus recommended by slimming clubs can be very expensive. If we don't achieve our goals we should adapt them and set further deadlines. The secret is not to give up, because of the numerous benefits associated with health improvement.

activity
INDIVIDUAL WORK
(2.4)

M2

D1

Use the table below to describe the problems you might face in trying to achieve your health improvement goals and why you should persevere!

Table 2.3

My health improvement goal	Problems I might face in sticking to my plan	The benefits to my health of achieving my goal
1		
2		
3		
4		

Hazards in Health and Social Care Environments and Health and Safety Legislation and Guidelines

keyword
Health and social care sector
The industry that provides a service to people with health and care needs.

This section describes some of the hazards found in the **health and social care sector**, their effects on the health and safety of people within those environments, and the responsibilities people have in controlling the hazards.It also builds on the information in the previous section, and looks at health and safety legislation and guidelines (laws, regulations) that aim to protect service users and health care workers.

Hazards in living and recreational areas include:

- faulty electrical appliances and switches, overloaded plug sockets, frayed flexes and power surges, which can cause fires, burns and electric shocks

- faulty gas appliances and gas leaks, which can cause fires and explosions, breathing problems, unconsciousness and death by asphyxiation (suffocation)

- water leaks. Rotten floorboards and floor coverings cause accidents and injury. In addition, when water comes into contact with electricity, there is a risk of fire and electrical injuries.

Electricity, gas and water are mains services. In the event of mains services' emergencies, health and care workers have a responsibility to switch or turn the services off and report the emergency to the mains supplier without delay.

Other fire hazards include:

- blocked fire exits and fire escape routes, and fire and smoke alarms that don't work or that people can't hear

- unsafe furnishings, such as cushions, loose and stretch covers, curtains and bedding, that don't display labels to show they are fire resistant

- open fires, cigarettes, cigars, pipes, lighters and matches.

The Management of Health and Safety at Work Regulations state that employers have a responsibility to train workers in fire prevention and procedures.

The Health and Safety at Work Act 1974 (HASWA) states that workers have a responsibility to report fire hazards to someone in authority without delay, to know emergency fire procedures and to prevent the risk of fire by working safely at all times.

Because many service users have mobility problems and sensory impairments, they are particularly at risk of health and safety hazards that cause slips, trips and falls. Accidents can cause cuts, bruises, sprains, strains and fractures (broken bones), as well as upset and distress. The following situations are most likely to cause accidents:

- poor working conditions, e.g. cramped, draughty working spaces with dim or harsh lighting, which affect the way health and care workers work together with service users

- poor building maintenance, e.g. loose handrails, chipped bathroom furniture, worn and slippery flooring, defective wiring and plumbing

- inappropriate furnishings, e.g. floor-length curtains, loose covers and rugs, all of which can make movement difficult.

The Management of Health and Safety at Work Regulations state that employers have a responsibility to:

- carry out risk assessments, identify and remove or reduce health and safety hazards

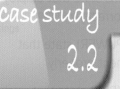

case study 2.2 — Working with hazardous substances

Lynne works with people with disabilities who need help to use the toilet. She is also responsible for keeping toilets clean and pleasant to use.

activity
GROUP WORK

(a) What hazardous substances would Lynne be working with?

(b) What health and safety risks are associated with these substances?

(c) Who is likely to be at risk?

(d) What steps should Lynne take to reduce the health and safety risks?

(e) What legislation affects how Lynne should work with hazardous substances?

(f) Why is it important that Lynne complies with health and safety legislation?

Infection control and food safety

Service users often have a low resistance to disease. Inadequate control of infectious diseases is a hazard because it leads to the spread of disease. Infectious diseases are usually caught from other people or from contaminated food.

Food Standards Agency www.foodstandards.gov.uk

The Management of Health and Safety at Work Regulations state that employers have a responsibility to train workers in infection control and food safety.

The Food Safety Act 1990 and the Food Safety (General Food Hygiene) Regulations state that workers have a responsibility to maintain:

■ a high standard of hygiene in areas where food is stored, prepared and cooked

■ a high standard of personal hygiene when handling food.

The Reporting of Injuries, Diseases and Dangerous Occurrences Regulations (RIDDOR) state that workers have a responsibility to report certain infectious diseases. Making reports is necessary to help prevent the spread of infectious disease.

Security

A lack of security measures is dangerous. Security measures protect people's safety, property and personal details, and prevent service users from leaving the building unless it is safe for them to do so. Inadequate personal safety precautions also put health and safety at risk. For example, workers who work alone and are unable to make contact with colleagues can feel isolated, be accused of things they haven't done and can be threatened or attacked.

> **remember**
>
> The vulnerability of service users means they are exposed to many health and safety hazards. Health and care workers have a responsibility to protect their health and safety by following safe work procedures which conform to the law.

The Health and Safety at Work Act 1974 (HASWA) states that workers have a responsibility to take care of their own security, the security of others and to report any security hazards to someone in authority straight away.

Throughout this section, reference has been made to the employer's responsibility to train workers.

Figure 2.14

Reasons why training is important

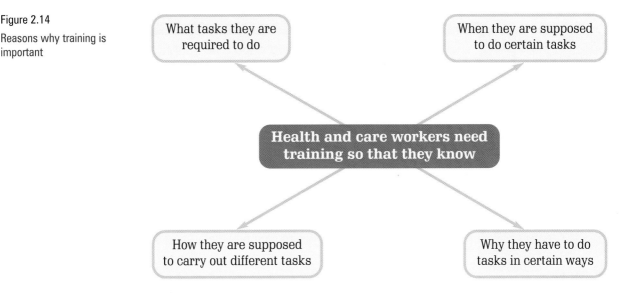

Health and care workers need training so that they know

- What tasks they are required to do
- When they are supposed to do certain tasks
- How they are supposed to carry out different tasks
- Why they have to do tasks in certain ways

Training

If health and care workers don't do their work properly because of poor staff training, they put their and service users' health and safety at risk.

The Health and Safety at Work Act 1974 states that workers must not carry out tasks for which they have not been trained. Therefore, all health and care workers must make the most of every training opportunity that presents itself. Training is an important part of professional development.

Health and care workers also need training in **manual handling**, for example turning someone over in bed or helping them move from their bed to a chair. If manual handling is not carried out safely, accidents happen. Thousands of injuries occur every year as a result of people moving awkward or heavy loads, many of which leave them unable to work again.

The Manual Handling Operations Regulations (MHOR) state that workers have a responsibility to follow workplace procedures for moving loads, which includes service users.

> **keyword**
>
> **Manual handling**
> Moving an object or load using the body as opposed to using a machine or equipment.

Links to Unit 3, pages 71–2.

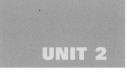

---

activity
GROUP WORK (2.5)

P4

Working in a group, survey your school, college or workplace and make a list of health and safety hazards that you see.

---

activity
GROUP WORK (2.6)

M3

D2

(a) Interview the person who has responsibility for health and safety at your school/college/workplace and find out what actions are taken to reduce risks.

(b) In your group, discuss the strengths and weaknesses of the actions taken to reduce risk and explain how they could be improved.

---

activity
INDIVIDUAL WORK (2.7)

P5

M4

Arrange a visit to a local health care provider, e.g. a GP practice, dental surgery, or to a local social care provider such as a residential home or luncheon club.

(a) Find out what health and safety legislation and guidelines the service provider has to follow.

(b) Produce a leaflet to be read by service users that describes the main points of the legislation and guidelines and explains why they have to be followed.

---

progress check

1. What are our everyday basic needs?
2. List four factors that can influence our health and needs.
3. Explain how these factors affect our health and needs.
4. What would you need to bear in mind when planning for improved health?
5. What might prevent someone sticking to their plan for improved health?
6. Why is it good for someone to achieve their health improvement goals?
7. Give six examples of hazards that might be found in a health or social care environment.
8. How are hazards in health or social care environments reduced?
9. What are the main laws and regulations that promote health and safety in health and care environments?
10. Explain why these laws and regulations need to be in place.

Books

Gresford, P. (1997), *Case Studies in Health and Social Care* (Heinemann)

Meggitt, C. (1997), *A Special Needs Handbook for Health and Social Care* (Hodder Arnold)

Michie, V. (2004), *Working in Care Settings* (Nelson Thornes)

Miller, J. (1996), *Social Care Practice* (Hodder and Stoughton)

Nolan, Y. (2003), *S/NVQ Level 2 in Care: Student Handbook* (Heinemann)

Owen Griffiths, A. (2005), *HACCP Works* (Highfield Publications)

Richards, A. (1999), *The Complete A–Z Health and Social Care Handbook* (Hodder Arnold)

Skelt, A. (1993), *Caring for People with Disabilities* (Pearson)

Sprenger, R. *The Foundation HACCP Handbook* (Highfield Publications)

Sprenger, R. and Fisher, I. *The Essentials of Health and Safety (Carers)* (Highfield Publications)

Windsor, G. and Moonie, N. (ed) (2000), *GNVQ Health and Social Care: Intermediate Compulsory Units with Edexcel Options* (Heinemann)

Leaflets

An Introduction to Health and Safety (HSE Books) available from www.hse.gov.uk

Other publications

Publications from the following organisations may be helpful:

Action on Smoking and Health (ASH); local drug action teams; local drug advisory services; health promotion units; first aid manuals; texts on home safety; The Royal Society for the Prevention of Accidents (RoSPA); National Advisory Committee on Nutritional Education (NACNE); Committee on Medical Aspects of Food Policy (COMA); Department of Health and the Joint Advisory Committee on Nutritional Education (JACNE).

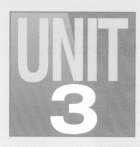

Vocational Experience in a Health or Social Care Setting

This unit covers:

- applying for work experience placement in a health or social care setting
- completing a period of work experience in a health or social care setting
- using interpersonal skills on work experience
- describing a period of work experience in a health or social care setting.

Completing a period of work experience in a health or social care setting will give you a valuable insight into the workplace and help you to develop both personally and as a worker. This unit describes examples of health and social care settings and how to apply for work experience. It describes interview skills and the interpersonal skills that you need to demonstrate during work experience. Finally, it directs you in producing evidence of your performance whilst on work experience and gives you an opportunity to think about how you have benefited from work experience and your suitability for a career in care work.

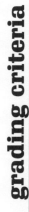

grading criteria

To achieve a **Pass** grade the evidence must show that the learner is able to:	To achieve a **Merit** grade the evidence must show that the learner is able to:	To achieve a **Distinction** grade the evidence must show that the learner is able to:
P1 use two different methods to present personal information for placement application Pg 60	**M1** describe strengths and weaknesses of own interpersonal skills as demonstrated on the work experience placement Pg 68	**D1** evaluate own work experience placement in terms of benefits to self and the placement Pg 75
P2 use appropriate interview skills for a health or social care work experience placement Pg 63	**M2** reflect on and review own performance on placement Pg 74	**D2** reflect on own personal attributes in relation to a career in health and social care Pg 75

grading criteria

To achieve a **Pass** grade the evidence must show that the learner is able to:	To achieve a **Merit** grade the evidence must show that the learner is able to:	To achieve a **Distinction** grade the evidence must show that the learner is able to:
P3 complete a period of work experience in a health or social care setting Pg 68		
P4 demonstrate the use of effective interpersonal skills on work experience Pg 68		
P5 complete a work experience diary or logbook Pg 68		

Applying for Work Experience Placement in a Health or Social Care Setting

People who work in health and social care must by law have had a satisfactory CRB check. This is a check made by the Criminal Records Bureau to identify whether someone is suitable to work with children and vulnerable adults. You must apply for a CRB check before you apply for a work placement.

Criminal Records Bureau www.crb.gov.uk

Methods of applying for work experience

When you apply for work experience, it is important that your application includes appropriate content. People who work in **health and social care settings** are very busy and don't have time to read or listen to information that is not relevant to their purpose. Your purpose is to obtain work experience. Your application must therefore only contain information that is appropriate to gaining work experience.

What should you include in an application for work experience?

- Your address and phone numbers: if you give a variety of contact details, people can choose a method of replying that fits in with their busy schedule.
- Your age and sex: these affect the activities you are allowed to carry out in health and social care settings.

keyword

Health and social care settings
The locations at which health and social care services are provided.

Figure 3.2
Dressing for an interview

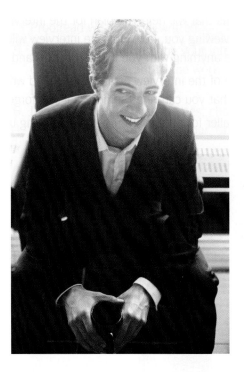

Interview skills

Rule number 1 – be punctual! Good timekeeping is essential in any workplace. If you're going to be late, telephone the organisation to explain why and organise another interview.

keyword

Social skills
Behaviours we need in order to socialise successfully with other people.

Personal skills
Behaviours that are part of our personalities.

remember

A careful application, preparing well and behaving appropriately during an interview are key to securing work experience.

Rule number 2 – use your **social** and **personal skills** to show you can relate to others! Health and social care workers need to have good social and personal skills and to be able to relate to other people. Make sure your mobile phone is turned off, smile, shake hands warmly with your interviewer and be courteous and respectful throughout the interview.

Rule number 3 – use positive communication skills. Unit 1 describes how to use verbal communication, body language and listening skills effectively.

Rule number 4 – answer questions clearly and confidently! Don't just answer with 'Yes' or 'No' but try to give full answers that show what you have learnt. Think before you speak and try to keep your voice steady. If you keep tripping up on your words, slow down and take a few deep breaths. If you make a mistake, correct yourself. Most importantly, be yourself and be positive!

Rule number 5 – ask questions! You may be asked at the end of the interview if you have any questions. Use this opportunity to find out more about the organisation, for example what people like about the work and what work you would be asked to do.

Figure 3.3
Interview questions

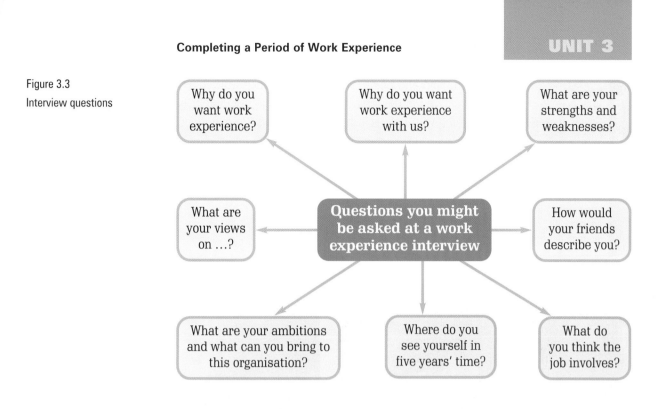

Why do you want work experience?

Why do you want work experience with us?

What are your strengths and weaknesses?

What are your views on …?

Questions you might be asked at a work experience interview

How would your friends describe you?

What are your ambitions and what can you bring to this organisation?

Where do you see yourself in five years' time?

What do you think the job involves?

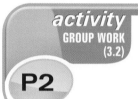

activity
GROUP WORK
(3.2)

P2

Work with a friend and take it in turns to role-play an interview for work experience. Give each other feedback on your interview skills and describe the ways in which you need to improve in order to be successful.

Completing a Period of Work Experience in a Health or Social Care Setting

Organisations that provide services to people with health and care needs fall into three main groups.

1. statutory organisations, which are in place because the law says they must exist

2. voluntary organisations (sometimes known as charities)

3. private organisations.

Statutory, voluntary and private **health and social care service providers** give formal care. Informal care is usually given by family, friends and neighbours.

You may have an idea of the type of health or social care organisation in which you would like to complete a period of work experience. However, having an

> **keyword**
>
> **Health and social care service providers**
> Organisations that meet the health and care needs of the public.

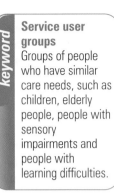

Service user groups
Groups of people who have similar care needs, such as children, elderly people, people with sensory impairments and people with learning difficulties.

open mind and being willing to experience work in a variety of settings will benefit you in the long run. For example, you might have your heart set on working with babies in a nursery setting. By experiencing work in other care settings you might realise you have skills and personality traits that make you more suited to working with other **service user groups**.

Figure 3.4

Different service user groups

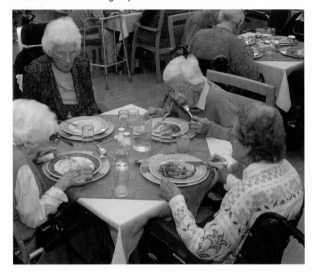
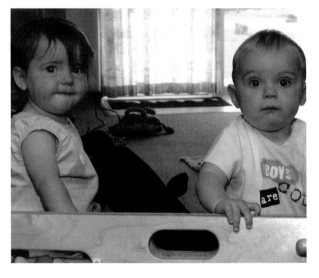

Statutory organisations

Examples of statutory organisations within the health and care sector:

- Primary health care services, which are the first point of contact that patients make with the health service. They include general practitioners (GPs), GP practice and community nurses, dentists, opticians, pharmacists, NHS walk-in centres and NHS Direct.

- Primary Care Trusts (PCTs), which work with local health and social care organisations to make sure that the community's health needs are met.

- Secondary health care services, which provide specialist health care. They include hospitals, the ambulance service and health care for people with a range of mental health needs.

- Local authority Social Service Departments, which assess whether someone in their area needs care and support. If they do, the Social Service Department works closely with other statutory service health and care providers to deliver the care and support that is needed.

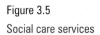
Figure 3.5
Social care services

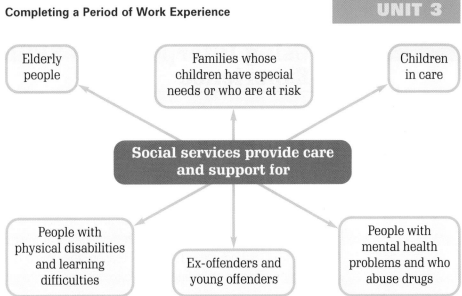

Voluntary organisations

There are many examples of voluntary organisations within the health and care sector.

Age Concern www.ageconcern.org.uk
Barnardo's www.barnardos.org.uk
Crisis www.crisis.org.uk
Scope www.scope.org.uk
The Terence Higgins Trust (THT) www.tht.org.uk

Private organisations

Examples of private organisations within the health and care sector:

- clinics and hospitals
- opticians
- dentists
- pharmacies
- residential care homes and agencies that provide care and support to people in their own homes
- child care providers
- shops, catalogues and Internet web sites.

Experience as many different care settings as possible. By doing so you will be in a position to make a sensible, informed choice about the type of organisation you want to be employed by and the service user group you want to work with.

remember

There are many organisations that provide health and social care services. Each has an important role to play in meeting service users' needs.

Using Interpersonal Skills on Work Experience

The communication cycle

You read in Unit 1 that understanding others, passing on information and making ourselves understood are key elements of the communication cycle. Communication barriers are caused by lack of understanding or failure to pass information on in ways that can be understood.

Good care practice requires health and care workers to understand the wants and needs of service users, the requirements of their work and to make themselves understood. For this reason, they must have excellent communication skills and be able to overcome communication barriers.

Links to Unit 1, page 3.

Skills

Good care practice also requires health and care workers to develop effective and appropriate relationships with the people they work with. In other words, they need to have excellent interpersonal skills. This section describes the communication and interpersonal skills that you need to demonstrate when on work experience. It also gives you an opportunity to identify how well you use your skills on work experience and to plan for their development.

You need to be able to interact with people in different ways, according to the situation and the people you are working with. You need to be able to interact effectively and appropriately:

- on a one-to-one basis
- within groups
- formally
- informally.

You need to be able to communicate effectively using:

- verbal communication
- body language, including the appropriate use of facial expressions and touch or contact.

You also need to know how to use words and body language to listen actively and focus on the individual, to show you are interested in them and want to understand what they are telling you.

Having an understanding of how to use proximity when relating to people is essential. Proximity is to do with closeness or nearness. We all have our own personal space. It is the area around our bodies which we like to keep private. Being physically close to someone can be a way of showing them support and understanding. However, entering someone's personal space without being invited is not acceptable and can cause offence. You need to know the extent of people's personal space and only enter when invited.

Figure 3.6
Active listening

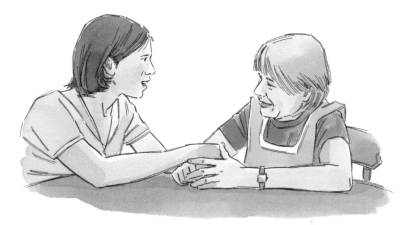

It is helpful to know how to overcome communication barriers that prevent people expressing themselves or understanding others. Unit 1 describes techniques for overcoming communication barriers.

You may be told personal information about service users. To protect their right to privacy and confidentiality, you must never pass this information on unless you have permission. For this reason, you need to demonstrate that you have respect for people and that you are trustworthy. Unit 1 describes how to maintain confidentiality of information.

Links to Unit 1, pages 13 and 25.

You need to be able to follow instructions. This is very important. People who can't or don't follow written or verbal instructions put others' health, safety and security at risk. They cannot be relied on and people lose confidence in them.

It is important to be well organised and good at timekeeping. Good timekeeping is essential in any workplace. People who are late for work, leave work early, take time off when it isn't necessary or who don't carry out activities when they should let others down, and are at risk of being sacked! On the other hand, people who have good timekeeping skills gain the respect of everyone they work with.

You need to be tactful, diplomatic and able to use discretion. This means being sensitive to people's feelings and situations, being able to make good judgements and behaving with consideration and maturity.

You need to be able to use your initiative. Using initiative is about doing things without needing to be asked. People who get on with jobs they've been trained to do without having to be prompted are worth their weight in gold. On the other hand, people who never do anything unless asked are irritating and make life hard for everyone else.

Health and care work is carried out by teams of people. You need to demonstrate teamwork skills, which include being:

- polite, honest, trustworthy and reliable
- keen to cooperate and get on with others
- willing to take responsibility for your own work activities and behaviour
- eager to learn new skills
- able to work accurately under pressure
- open to suggestions and feedback.

remember

Work in health and social care is about effective communication and developing relationships with people. For this reason, health and care workers must have excellent interpersonal skills. Be aware of your strengths so that you can build on them, and your weaknesses so that you can overcome them.

Learndirect Advice includes information on careers, job profiles, interview skills, etc. www.learndirect-advice.co.uk

Information on careers in the National Health Service www.nhscareers.nhs.uk

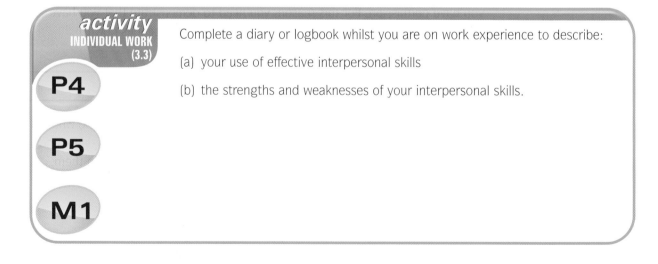

activity
INDIVIDUAL WORK (3.3)

P4

P5

M1

Complete a diary or logbook whilst you are on work experience to describe:

(a) your use of effective interpersonal skills

(b) the strengths and weaknesses of your interpersonal skills.

Describing a Period of Work Experience in a Health or Social Care Setting

keyword

Informed choice
A choice based on knowledge and understanding.

keyword

Multiculturalism
A principle that encourages people from different cultural backgrounds to live and work together and benefit from each other's lifestyles and experiences.

Work–life balance
A healthy balance between work time and personal time.

The organisation

Finding out about different health and social care organisations will help you make an **informed choice** about where you want to begin your career. For example, you might find it useful to know:

■ whether they are in the statutory, voluntary or private sector

■ what services they provide and the service user groups they work with

■ their principles (values and beliefs) about **multiculturalism** and **work–life balance**, etc.

■ their reputation for health and safety

■ the work that people do and the opportunities for career progression.

Find out how your work experience organisations are funded, e.g. does their income come from:

■ social insurance (taxes levied by the Government)?

■ charges made to service users?

■ Public-Private Partnerships (PPPs), i.e. partnerships between the Government and private organisations?

■ grants or the National Lottery?

■ fund-raising events?

Funding is used to buy and maintain the resources an organisation needs in order to provide services.

Figure 3.7
Resources

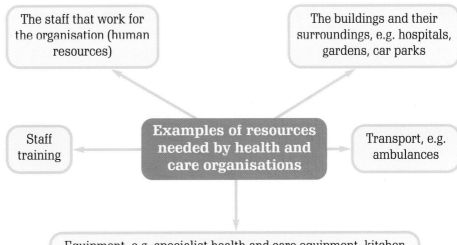

Knowing how an organisation is funded will help you understand why there may be problems with resources, for example services that don't meet people's expectations, services that have to be withdrawn, and staff shortages.

Policies are official documents that describe an organisation's responsibilities when providing services. For example, an organisation's health and safety policy describes its responsibilities in obeying health and safety legislation. Procedures are based on the organisation's policies and tell workers how to carry out their activities. For example, health and safety procedures describe exactly how to carry out hazardous activities.

Health and care workers have a responsibility to know the policies and procedures that affect their work. Find out where policies and procedures are kept at your work experience organisation and use your time productively by getting to know the ones that affect your activities.

Links to Unit 4, page 99.

The staff

It's interesting and useful to find out about issues relating to staff in health and care organisations. Learning about their roles and responsibilities, the skills, qualifications and personal qualities needed for different job roles, training and opportunities for career development, and employment terms and conditions will help you make an informed choice about where you want to begin your career.

If service users' needs are to be met, it's very important that health and care workers know their **job roles** and **responsibilities** and the roles and responsibilities of the people they work with.

Find out the roles and responsibilities of the people at your work placement. Sources of information you could use include workers themselves, their job descriptions and health and care books, journals, magazines and websites.

If you plan to make a career in health or social care, you will need to develop appropriate skills and personal attributes (qualities). You looked earlier at the communication and interpersonal skills needed by health and care workers. Other skills needed for working in health and care include:

- domestic skills; these are very important, and people who, for example, willingly clean and shop are worth their weight in gold
- maintaining health, safety and security
- care skills such as helping service users with their personal care and providing emotional, physical, social and intellectual support.

Professional development

Health and care workers must be willing to undergo continuous professional development (CPD), i.e. to continually update workplace skills and learning and gain relevant qualifications. There are many ways that health and care workers can develop their skills and achieve qualifications:

keyword

Job role
What a job is all about, e.g. cleaning.

Responsibility
The duties or tasks that are part of the job role, e.g. hoovering, dusting, washing windows.

- informal learning, such as work shadowing, reading specialist magazines and journals, watching educational TV programmes, videos and DVDs, and checking out care-related websites
- formal learning, such as attending training sessions and studying courses delivered by colleges of further education, local education authorities, independent training providers, distance learning providers and Internet learning providers.

Figure 3.8
Continuous professional development

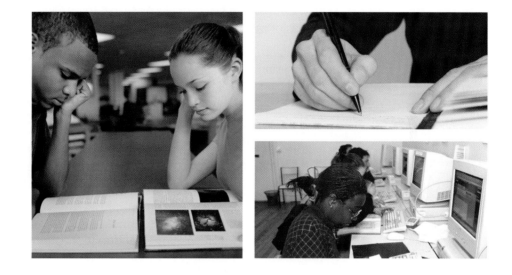

Formal learning usually leads to a qualification, such as Basic First Aid, BTEC First Diploma in Health and Social Care and NVQ in Health and Social Care. However, informal learning is just as important because it provides much of the knowledge and understanding needed to gain a qualification.

Talk to the people you meet on work placement and find out what skills, personal attributes and qualifications they need to do their jobs and how they have developed them. Knowing what is required for different jobs can help you make an informed choice about where you see yourself working in the future.

Induction

All new health and social care workers have to take part in an induction process. During induction, health care workers are expected to develop an understanding of a wide range of topics, including:

- health and safety, e.g. safe moving and handling techniques, fire training, how to work with hazardous substances and infection control
- how to support people with personal hygiene and oral care
- the prevention and care of **pressure ulcers**
- **continence** and bladder care
- food and nutrition

keyword

Pressure ulcers
Wounds caused by pressure or friction.

Continence
Control of the bladder and bowel.

71

- privacy, dignity, diversity and equality
- customer service and how to deal with aggression.

They are also expected to learn how to make simple measurements, such as temperature, blood pressure, pulse and respiration.

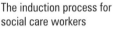

Links to Unit 2, page 51.

During induction, social care workers have to develop an understanding of six key areas of care.

Figure 3.9

The induction process for social care workers

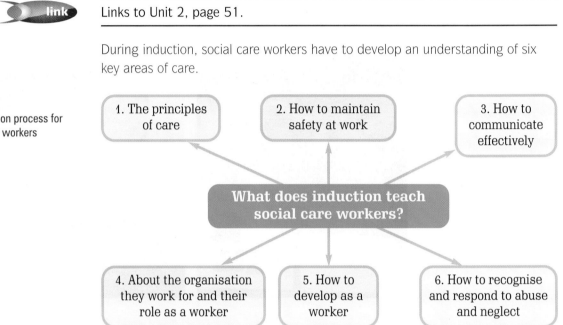

Monitoring performance

The main role of a supervisor is to monitor the performance of staff and give them feedback about their performance. Feedback can be given both on the job and in private, for example during appraisals. One of the purposes of feedback sessions is to agree a plan that records a worker's continuing professional development needs and how and when they will be met.

Find out how your work experience organisations monitor staff performance and how they meet needs for CPD. Knowing how performance is monitored and how an organisation supports the development of its staff can help you make an informed choice about whether you want to work for it in the future.

Terms and conditions

An organisation's employment terms and conditions are important because they form the basis on which staff are employed. They are usually written into contracts of employment and describe:

- pay details, e.g. pay scales and how often wages or salaries are paid
- hours of work, including lunch times
- holiday details
- pension details

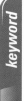

Probationary period
The period of time during which a new member of staff is monitored to see if they and the job are right for each other.

- employment benefits, e.g. training opportunities
- details of **probationary periods**.

Check out the terms and conditions at your work experience organisation. Talk to staff to find out if they are satisfied with their terms and conditions. Information like this can help you make an informed decision about whether you would like to be employed by the organisation.

Your own performance

You read above that health and care workers are required to undergo continuous professional development (CPD) throughout their career. This includes:

Career development plan
An action plan that shows how you aim to move forward in your career.

- reflecting on (thinking about) and reviewing (assessing) their knowledge and skills
- producing **career development plans** which record their strengths and weaknesses and describe how their knowledge and skills need to be developed and improved
- developing their strengths and improving their weaknesses.

case study 3.1 — The new girl

Sue is new to care work. She has been asked to run a quiz for seven or eight elderly and disabled residents, some of whom have communication difficulties and memory problems.

The quiz is a dismal failure. None of the residents enjoys it and none feels a sense of achievement for having taken part in it. Rumour spreads that 'the new girl is useless'.

activity — GROUP WORK

(a) What does Sue need to do first?

(b) How could she improve the way she carries out the activity?

(c) How could she assess whether the changes she makes are an improvement?

This section aims to direct you in your development whilst on work experience and give you an opportunity to identify how well you perform and evaluate the benefits of work experience.

You read earlier about the importance of good timekeeping, being able to follow instructions and using your initiative. Using feedback from the people you work with will help you reflect on and review how well you perform in these areas and plan for improvement.

You should also reflect on how you perform the activities you undertake. For example, how do you use the Care Value Base when working with service users? Do you demonstrate respect for their privacy, dignity, diversity and equality? Do you maintain the confidentiality of their personal information?

How do you maintain health, safety and security? Do you know and follow safe working procedures at all times? And how effectively do you meet service users':

- physical care needs, e.g. to move around, eat and drink?
- emotional care needs, e.g. for patience and understanding?
- intellectual care needs, e.g. for stimulating conversation?
- social care needs, e.g. for staying in contact with family and friends?
- personal care needs, e.g. personal hygiene, dressing and grooming?

Health and care activities require a multitude of skills and you won't be expected to know everything in the first few weeks of your work experience! Continually reflect on and review the knowledge and skills you gain and ask the people you work with for feedback on your performance. If there are any weaknesses in the way you do your work, talk with your supervisor about how you can improve, for example by participating in career progression opportunities such as work shadowing, on-the-job training and training courses.

As your learning and skills improve, the more confident you will become and, as your self-confidence grows, you will become more effective at your job and more valued and respected by the people you work with.

> **remember**
>
> Work experience offers countless opportunities for learning, both about work in a health and social care setting and about yourself. Enjoy your work placements and make the most of every learning opportunity that presents itself!

activity
INDIVIDUAL WORK (3.4)

M2

Reflect on and review your performance on work experience. Use your work experience diary or logbook to record your performance strengths and weaknesses and to describe how you can improve your performance.

activity
INDIVIDUAL WORK (3.5)

D1

Sum up the benefits of your work experience for:

(a) you

(b) your work experience organisation.

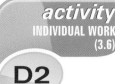

activity
INDIVIDUAL WORK (3.6)

D2

In what ways do you think you are suited to a career as a health or care worker? Explain your answer.

progress check

1. Give three examples of how you can apply for a work experience placement.

2. Explain how to use the telephone effectively.

3. Describe how you would prepare for an interview for work experience.

4. Give five examples of good interview skills.

5. Give three examples of interpersonal skills that health and care workers need to develop and use.

6. Give three examples of caring skills that health and care workers need to develop and use.

7. Describe the skills and personal qualities needed by people who work in teams.

8. Why is it important that health and care workers constantly reflect on and review their interpersonal skills and performance?

9. Why is it important that health and care workers seek feedback from the people they work with about their interpersonal skills and performance?

10. Describe five factors that would help you decide which health or social care organisation you would like to work for.

Books

Barratt, C. (2000), *Intermediate Health and Social Care* (Oxford University Press)

Burnard, P. and Morrison, P. (1997), *Caring and Communicating* (Palgrave Macmillan)

Department for Education and Skills, *Skills for Life, Teachers' Reference Pack, Social Care* (DfES)

Michie, V. (2004), *Working in Care Settings* (Nelson Thornes)

Miller, J. (1996), *Social Care Practice* (Hodder and Stoughton)

Nazarko, L. (2000), *NVQs in Nursing and Residential Homes* (Blackwell Publishing)

Pearce, R. (2003), *Profiles and Portfolios of Evidence* (Nelson Thornes)
Skelt, A. (1993), *Caring for People with Disabilities* (Pearson)
Wallis, J. (2001), *Health Care* (Heinemann)

Leaflets

The Right Start – Work Experience for Young People: Health and Safety Basics for Employers (Health and Safety Executive) available from www.hse.gov.uk

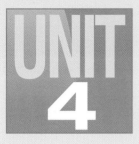

UNIT 4

Cultural Diversity in Health and Social Care

This unit covers:

- the diversity of individuals in society
- practices in different religious or secular beliefs
- factors that influence the equality of opportunity for individuals in society
- the rights of individuals in health and social care environments.

There is a huge diversity of individuals in British society, in particular a wide range of social and political differences and differences in religious and secular (non-religious) beliefs. These differences are reflected in the groups of people who use health and social care services. For this reason, health and social care workers need to understand diversity and how diversity affects the services they provide. They also need to understand the moral and legal rights of the people they work with, their responsibilities in supporting and protecting people's rights, and how their understanding of diversity can be used to promote equal opportunities and to help those they work with feel valued.

grading criteria

To achieve a **Pass** grade the evidence must show that the learner is able to:	To achieve a **Merit** grade the evidence must show that the learner is able to:	To achieve a **Distinction** grade the evidence must show that the learner is able to:
P1 describe social and political factors that make people different from each other Pg 80	**M1** explain differences in health and social care service delivery necessary to promote equality of opportunity for individuals Pg 92	**D1** explain the possible effects of discrimination on the physical, intellectual, emotional, and social health/well-being of individuals Pg 96
P2 compare the practices and beliefs of individuals from two contrasting religious groups/secular beliefs Pg 80	**M2** identify discriminatory practice and suggest how it can be avoided Pg 94	**D2** evaluate the effectiveness of the chosen legislation and code of practice/charter in valuing diversity, promoting equality and supporting the rights of individuals in health and social care environments Pg 102

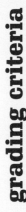

To achieve a **Pass** grade the evidence must show that the learner is able to:	To achieve a **Merit** grade the evidence must show that the learner is able to:	To achieve a **Distinction** grade the evidence must show that the learner is able to:
P3 describe factors that may influence the equality of opportunities for individuals Pg 92	**M3** explain how the legislation and code of practice/charter supports the rights of individuals within the chosen environment Pg 102	
P4 identify how understanding diversity can help promote the rights of patients/service users Pg 102		
P5 describe one piece of relevant legislation and one code of practice or charter for a chosen health or social care environment that aims to support the rights of the individual Pg 102		

The Diversity of Individuals in Society

Social and political diversity

Social and political **diversity** is to do with the differences between individuals and the differences between groups of people.

Ethnicity

Everyone has an ethnicity. People who have the same ethnic background share, to one degree or another, the same history, religion, language, birthplace and physical appearance. Unit 1 shows the different ethnic groups in Britain in 2001. Plans are being made to hold the next census in 2011.

www.statistics.gov.uk/census

Social class

British society has a number of different social classes. The most common way of deciding someone's social class is by their occupation or job. Unit 1 shows how people in Britain are classed according to their occupation.

www.statistics.gov.uk/methods_quality/ns_sec

Links to Unit 1, pages 14–15.

Gender and sexuality

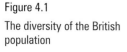

Socialisation
The process of rearing children to think and behave in the ways that their family and society expects of them.

Gender is to do with femininity and masculinity. When a baby is born, it has no gender. It acquires its gender as it grows up and is **socialised** by the society it lives in. Different people have different ideas about what makes for masculinity and femininity. For example, some men behave in what you might call a feminine way – they are house husbands and look after the children and the home. And some women behave in what you might call a masculine way – they are tough, assertive and competitive.

Some men and women are uncomfortable with their gender and the way others expect them to think and behave. Transsexuals behave as if they were of the opposite sex and others undergo treatment or surgery to change their sex.

Our sex is determined by our genitals (sex organs). Most of us are born male or female although some people are born 'intersex', i.e. their sex organs are not distinct, which makes it difficult to tell whether they are a boy or a girl. Our sexuality is to do with our sexual preference for other people. Unit 1 describes sexuality and sexual preference.

Age

British society is populated by people of different ages, e.g. children, youths, young adults, adults, middle-aged people and elderly people. A mixture of age groups allows society to benefit from the energy and enthusiasm of youth and the experience and wisdom of maturity and old age.

Figure 4.1

The diversity of the British population

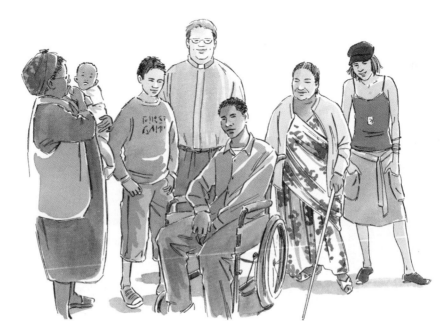

Family structure

Differences in family structure also contribute to the diversity of British society. Unit 1 describes the different types of families in Britain today.

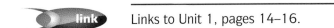

Links to Unit 1, pages 14–16.

You may find the following information useful:

- There are currently (2006) about 1.8 million single-parent families in Britain, which is a quarter of all families, and they care for 3 million children.
- In 2003/04, one in six adults aged 16 and over in Great Britain lived alone.
- In England in spring 2004, 58 per cent of young men aged 20 to 24, and 39 per cent of young women of the same age, lived at home with their parents.
- There were 306,000 marriages in the UK in 2003 and 167,000 divorces.

Disability

A report published in 2005 by the Social Exclusion Unit that looked at disability stated that:

- there are 5.9 million people of working age in Britain who are disabled
- one in three people in Britain has a long-term ill health condition
- 80 per cent of people experience a year of being disabled at some point in their lives.

These figures demonstrate that large numbers of us are ill or disabled.

- Physical ill health includes chest, heart and circulatory problems and disabilities such as sensory impairments and mobility problems.
- Mental ill health includes depression, **dementia** and Alzheimer's disease (a form of dementia).
- Learning difficulties that are disabling in one way or another include Down's syndrome and **autism**.

keyword

Dementia
A condition which causes memory loss, confusion and loss of mental ability and social skills.

keyword

Autism
A disorder in which people are unable to interact with others.

Religious and secular beliefs

Beliefs are ideas or principles that we believe in and think of as true. People living in Britain hold a wide range of religious and secular beliefs. They include atheists, Buddhists, Christians, Hindus, Humanists, Jehovah's Witnesses, Jews, Muslims, Pagans, Rastafarians and Sikhs. You will read more about religious and secular beliefs shortly.

remember

We are all different and our differences contribute to the rich diversity of the British population.

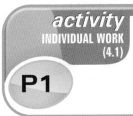

activity
INDIVIDUAL WORK
(4.1)

P1

Describe how you and the people you live, study, work and socialise with are different from each other.

Think about ethnic background, social class, gender, sexuality, age, family structure, disability and religious and secular beliefs.

Practices in Different Religious or Secular Beliefs

In order to care for people appropriately, health and care workers need to understand how service users' religious and secular beliefs affect their needs and preferences. This section describes some of these beliefs and the forms of worship and festivals practised by different people. It also describes some of their dietary needs and health and medical beliefs. Remember, though, that the practices and needs of people who share a belief can be as varied as those of people who have different beliefs.

 Links to Unit 2, page 38.

i www.bbc.co.uk/religion
www.ethnicityonline.net
www.multiculturalcalendar.com

Atheism

Atheists deny that God exists.

Figure 4.2

Reasons why people don't believe in God

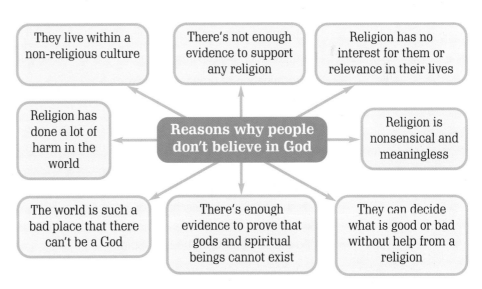

Atheists usually have non-religious ceremonies for weddings and funerals, and some atheists have special ceremonies for naming babies. They don't have particular beliefs and practices regarding diet, health and medicine.

Buddhism

Buddhism is a way of life based on the teachings of Buddha. Buddha taught that people can overcome suffering by living a life filled with good behaviour, happiness and compassion.

Buddhists worship in a temple or at home, where they meditate, chant, say prayers and listen to religious readings. There are no set times for worship – people worship when it suits them to do so.

Buddhists believe in reincarnation, which is a cycle of birth, life, death and rebirth; and in karma, which is to do with how their behaviour in previous lives affects them now and in the future. In other words, they believe that you reap what you sow.

The main Buddhist festivals are:

- the Wesak or 'Festival of Light', which celebrates Buddha's enlightenment, when he was released from the cycle of reincarnation
- Dharma Day, which celebrates Buddha's teachings
- Sangha Day, which celebrates the spiritual community
- Parinirvana Day, which marks the day that Buddha died and reached his nirvana (paradise or heaven).

There are no Buddhist laws regarding diet. However, because they are not supposed to be responsible for the death of living things, many Buddhists are vegetarians or **vegans**. And many don't drink alcohol because it dulls the mind.

Buddhist health and medical beliefs are based on the teachings of Buddha. Many Buddhists believe that:

- taking medication that contains animal products or alcohol is wrong
- meditation and chanting can be used to relieve pain
- termination of pregnancy is wrong
- dying is nothing to be frightened of
- it takes at least three days for consciousness to leave a body, so dead bodies should not be disturbed by, for example, a post mortem during that time.

keyword

Vegans
People who don't eat meat and animal products, such as milk and eggs

Christianity

Christians follow the teachings of Jesus Christ. He taught that there is only one God but that God consists of three 'persons' or the 'Holy Trinity': God the Father, God the Son and God the Holy Spirit.

Christians worship God in church services, usually on Sundays. They pray, sing hymns and listen to readings from the Bible, which is the Christian holy book. Jesus's last supper on earth is remembered in the Eucharist (Holy Communion) service, when bread and wine are eaten which Christians believe represent Jesus's body and blood.

The most important Christian festivals are:

- Christmas Day, when Jesus was born
- Good Friday, when Jesus was crucified (put to death on the cross) to save Christians from the consequences of their sins

- Easter Sunday, when Jesus rose from the dead (the Resurrection)
- Ascension Day, when Jesus ascended (rose) into heaven to join God
- Pentecost, when the Holy Spirit came down to earth from heaven and the Christian Church began.

Christians aren't expected to eat a specific diet. However, some don't eat meat on Fridays, others **fast** before taking the Eucharist, and some don't drink alcohol.

Christians have a range of health and medical beliefs, for example many:

- won't take medication that contains alcohol
- believe that it is good for them to suffer pain
- don't agree with contraception
- oppose termination of pregnancy unless the mother's life is at risk
- believe that prayers will help them on their way to heaven and so might want to be visited by a priest when they are dying.

> **keyword**
>
> **Fast**
> To give up food and drink temporarily.

Hinduism

People who follow Hinduism are known as Hindus. Hindus believe in one God (Brahman), but they also worship many deities who represent different aspects of Brahman, such as Brahma (the creator), Vishnu (the preserver) and Shiva (the destroyer). Like Buddhists, they believe in reincarnation and karma.

Hindus believe that living a good life is more important than religious ritual and worship. The Vedas (Hindu scriptures) teach Hindus how to live, through parables, stories and legends.

The most widely celebrated Hindu festival is Diwali or the 'Festival of Lights'. It is thought to be the start of the new year and celebrates the triumph of light (knowledge) over darkness (ignorance).

Hindus are not supposed to harm any living thing, so most eat a strict vegetarian diet. In addition:

- many believe the cow is sacred so won't eat beef or anything that contains beef products
- some won't drink alcohol
- some fast on specials occasions, such as holy days.

Hindus have a variety of health and medical beliefs, for example many:

- believe that traditional foods and **Ayurvedic medicine** have the power to heal
- won't take medication that contains animal products
- oppose termination of pregnancy unless the mother's life is at risk .

> **keyword**
>
> **Ayurvedic medicine**
> A system of diet, exercise, meditation and herbal remedies that is used to treat imbalances in the body.

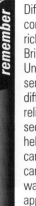

Sikhs have a number of different health and medical beliefs, for example:

■ medication must be vegetarian or not contain any pork or beef products

■ some refuse pain relief as they prefer to use pain as a learning experience

■ most have a deep sense of modesty. Physical examinations must be carried out by a member of the same sex

■ cleanliness is very important. They must wash their hair, which they never cut, frequently and bathe in running water if possible

■ sex before and outside of marriage is forbidden

■ termination of pregnancy is not allowed unless the mother's life is in danger

■ human life is sacred but the dead body is not.

case study 4.1 Meeting religious and secular needs

A new community centre is being planned for an inner city location. The centre will be staffed by, and provide day care and support for, people with a range of different religious and secular beliefs.

activity
GROUP WORK

Describe, using examples, factors that:

(a) the architects will have to take into account when designing the centre

(b) the manager will have to take into account when employing staff and planning work rotas and holidays

(c) the kitchen staff will have to consider when buying, preparing and cooking food

(d) the care workers will have to consider when organising transport to and from the centre, trips out, social events and recreational activities

(e) the health and care workers will have to consider when giving medical and personal care and support to people who are living at the centre.

activity
INDIVIDUAL WORK
(4.2)

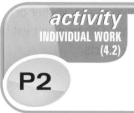

P2

Talk to a couple of friends or colleagues who have different religious/secular beliefs. Write an article for a newspaper, for example, that compares each person's different practices and beliefs.

Factors that Influence the Equality of Opportunity for Individuals in Society

Social and political factors that influence equal opportunity

Equal opportunity is about everyone having access to the same opportunities. However, our social and political differences mean that we don't all have equal opportunities, as the following examples illustrate.

Equal Opportunities Commission www.eoc.org.uk

Table 4.1

Social and political factors	Examples of how social and political factors influence equal opportunities
Ethnicity	Many people from different ethnic backgrounds can't read, understand or speak English. As a result, they don't have the same opportunity to access health and care services as people who use English.
Religious beliefs	People with different religious beliefs may have specific dietary needs. Organisations which don't offer menus that take different beliefs into account deny people the same opportunity as others to have their dietary needs met.
Social class	People in the lower social classes are more likely to earn low wages or be dependent on benefits. For this reason they don't have the same opportunity as people higher up the social ladder to buy themselves a healthy lifestyle.
Gender	Many people believe that caring for dependent relatives is a feminine role. This traditional belief can deny women the opportunity to develop themselves in the world of work and men the opportunity to be fulfilled as carers.
Sexuality	Many jobs are closed to people who are gay or lesbian, usually because of other people's homophobic attitudes. Denying homosexuals employment denies them the same opportunities that heterosexuals enjoy.
Age	Older people are knowledgeable, experienced and wise. However, they are less likely to be asked for their opinions than younger people, and, as a result, are not given the same opportunities to have their say.
Family structure	Family structure can affect people's ability to make the most of opportunities that are open to everyone else: e.g. elderly people who live alone and lone carers find it hard to access services and play a role in their communities.
Disability	People with disabilities are denied many opportunities to which healthy, able-bodied people have access: e.g. wheelchair users have restricted access to public transport; people with mental health problems may be denied employment, and people with learning difficulties can find it difficult to be accepted within a community.

As these examples show, differences create disadvantage. Disadvantaged people need help and support to access opportunities that the rest of us take for granted. For this reason, equal opportunity is also about providing help and support to people, so that they can access opportunities and be treated as fairly as everybody else.

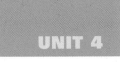
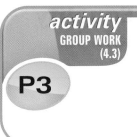

Talk with four or five friends and family members about the opportunities you each have in life, for example to be educated, use health care services, practise your religion, use public transport, be employed, have a social life, start a family, etc. Compare the extent to which each of you is able to access these opportunities and describe the factors that affect your access to equal opportunities.

Produce a display about two health or social care settings of your choice, such as a luncheon club for infirm, elderly people, a residential home for people with learning difficulties or sensory impairments, a drop-in centre for teenage parents and their children, that:

(a) compares the different ways that service users' needs and preferences are met

(b) explains how the services provided promote equal opportunities.

Discriminatory practice

As you read in Unit 1, discriminatory practice happens when people let their negative prejudices and the way they stereotype and label others affect their behaviour. People who knowingly practise discrimination are bullies and the people they bully are usually different from them, weaker and more vulnerable. Discrimination and bullying are unfair and can stop people having access to opportunities that others enjoy.

Service users are vulnerable. Health and care workers have a responsibility to help them access opportunities that will meet their wants, preferences and needs. If a worker's negative beliefs and attitudes affect the way they work, service users' needs will not be met in an appropriate and acceptable way.

Links to Unit 1, pages 19–21.

Non-discriminatory work practice

Non-discriminatory work practice is work practice that treats people fairly and promotes equal opportunities. You read in Unit 1 about the legislation that aims to protect people from discrimination and promote equal opportunities. You also read about the professional codes of practice and charters that describe the standards that workers are expected to follow in their activities.

Institutions or organisations that provide services, including providers of health and social care, have a responsibility to comply with anti-discriminatory legislation and professional codes of practice and charters. They do this by writing anti-discriminatory policies and procedures, which describe how the organisation and its staff aim to treat people fairly and how victims of discrimination can have their complaints dealt with.

Health and care organisations also write their own care charters, which tell service users how their rights to equal opportunities and fair treatment are fostered and promoted.

Health and social care workers have a duty to promote non-discriminatory work practice in their day-to-day work. They can do this by:

- following non-discriminatory work procedures and codes of practice
- being friendly and approachable with everyone, regardless of their differences
- being interested in people and finding out how their backgrounds affect their care needs and preferences
- reporting any concerns they have about discriminatory behaviour to a supervisor or manager
- reflecting on their own behaviour. They should ask themselves whether they label and stereotype people, whether they let their prejudices cause them to treat some people less favourably than others, and whether they use expressions and laugh at jokes that could be hurtful or offensive. They should also ask for feedback about their work practice from the people they work with, and act on feedback if it will improve their work practice.

Health and social care workers can also help those they work with to learn about and recognise the value of people's differences. Ways to do this include:

- putting up visual displays that show positive images of people's differences, e.g. ethnic diversity, gender, age and disability
- organising activities, such as visits and discussion groups, that will increase people's understanding of one another
- tactfully making colleagues and service users aware of their discriminatory behaviour, even if it is unintended and accidental.

Supporting people's rights to fair and equal treatment, having a positive approach and understanding why people think, feel and behave as they do ensures that everyone feels valued and respected, regardless of their differences. And it ensures that service users are cared for in ways that meet their individual needs and preferences.

 Links to Unit 1, pages 17–8 and 21–5.

case study 4.2 — Discriminatory work practice

Fairways is a residential care home for elderly people. The residents have a range of care needs, including those caused by dementia, sight and hearing impairments and mobility problems.

Geraldine has just started work at Fairways. She has never worked in care before. You have heard her talking about the residents as 'wrinklies', 'cloth ears', 'old bats' and 'psychos'. She shouts at everyone and tries to do everything for them, for example feed and dress them. Some of the residents are incontinent and others don't have a good grasp of English. She avoids working with these people on the grounds that having to change continence pads disgusts her and that 'if people choose to live in England, they should jolly well learn the language'.

activity
INDIVIDUAL WORK

(a) In what ways is Geraldine's work practice discriminatory?

(b) How could Geraldine be helped to work in an anti-discriminatory way?

activity
INDIVIDUAL WORK (4.5)

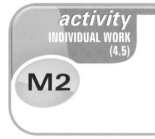

M2

(a) Observe the way that people at your school/college/workplace talk about and behave with each other and identify examples of discriminatory practice.

(b) Write a short report for your teacher/tutor/manager, in which you make them aware of the discriminatory practice and make recommendations as to how it can be avoided.

Figure 4.6
Not good practice…

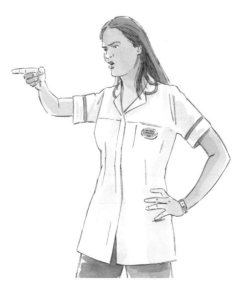

The effects of discrimination

As well as denying people access to equal opportunities, discrimination can have tragic effects on people's health and well-being.

Figure 4.7

How does discrimination affect people?

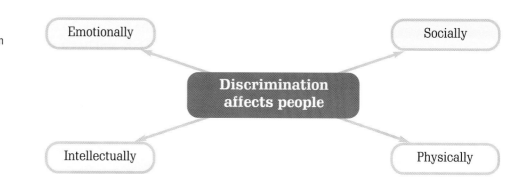

The emotional effects of discrimination include:

- anger and resentment because the treatment is wrong and unfair
- fear because of being intimidated and bullied
- stress and depression
- loss of self-confidence and self-worth.

The social effects of discrimination include **isolation** and **social exclusion**, which lead to loneliness and breakdown of relationships. Loneliness, depression and low self-confidence and self-worth make it difficult to build new relationships.

Discrimination can also have intellectual effects. Depression, social exclusion and low self-confidence and self-worth can stop people communicating, learning and developing skills, which makes it difficult for them to find work. As a result, people who suffer discrimination are unlikely to achieve fulfilment through employment or to be able to afford a good quality of life.

The emotional, social and intellectual effects of discrimination have physical effects on people's health. For example, they may not look after their personal hygiene or eat properly, and they may smoke, drink or take drugs in an attempt to deal with their feelings. As a result, they may develop physical ill health conditions and not be able to maintain their standard of living. They begin to be **deprived**.

Children growing up in deprivation suffer poor physical and mental health. They miss out on schooling and don't develop the skills necessary to get a job. As a result, as adults they live in poverty and their own children grow up in deprivation.

keyword

Isolation
Being alone, lacking companionship.

Social exclusion
Being left out, not allowed to join in.

keyword

Deprived
Disadvantaged, underprivileged.

Table 4.2

Conventions, legislation and regulations...	... and their purpose
The Equal Pay Act 1970 The Sex Discrimination Act 1975 The Race Relations Act 1976 The Disability Discrimination Act 1995 The Human Rights Act 1998	These protect us from unfair treatment and discrimination.
The European Convention on Human Rights and Fundamental Freedoms 1950 The Convention on the Rights of the Child 1989	These conventions describe everyone's basic human rights to: • life, freedom and security • food, health and housing • education and work • protection of private life and property • freedom of expression, thought and belief • a fair trial and freedom from torture • freedom from discrimination on any grounds.
The Children Act 2004	This protects children's rights by giving local authorities flexibility in the way they meet children's needs, including children with special needs.
The Mental Health Act 1983	This protects the rights of the general public by compulsorily hospitalising people with severe mental health problems. It also protects the rights of the patient by explaining: • who is involved in the decision for them to be hospitalised • the patient's or the patient's nearest relative's right of appeal.
The Care Standards Act 2000	This protects vulnerable people's right to the highest possible standard of care. • Care providers must provide care in ways that meet the National Care Standards. The care they give is monitored by the Commission for Social Care Inspection and the Healthcare Commission. • People's suitability to work in care must be checked and workers must be trained to do their jobs. Checks and training are monitored by the Social Care Councils for England, Wales, Northern Ireland and Scotland.
The NHS and Community Care Act 1990	This protects the rights of older and disabled people to be cared for at home and in the community in ways that take account of their choices.
The Residential Care and Nursing Homes Regulations 2002	This protects the right of people living in care homes to be protected from danger and harm.
The Data Protection Act 1998	This gives people the right to check what information is held about them. It also tells organisations how they can use and store information so that it remains confidential.

Health Care Commission www.healthcarecommission.org.uk
Commission for Social Care Inspection www.csci.org.uk
General Social Care Council www.gscc.org.uk
Care Council for Wales www.ccwales.org.uk
Northern Ireland Social Care Council www.niscc.info
Scottish Social Services Council www.sssc.uk.com

Codes of practice and charters

The General Social Care Council for England, the Care Council for Wales, the Northern Ireland Social Care Council and the Scottish Social Services Council have codes of practice that spell out the standards of care practice expected from everyone working in social care. The aim of the codes of practice is to improve work practice, which in turn improves protection for service users' rights. Social care employers and registered social care workers who break the codes deny service users their rights. They may be removed from the Social Care Register.

The codes of practice say that social care employers must:

■ check that people are suitable to be employed and understand their roles and responsibilities

■ write policies and procedures that enable social care workers to meet the Code of Practice for Social Care Workers

■ provide training and development to help social care workers improve their skills and knowledge

■ write policies and procedures that deal with dangerous, discriminatory behaviour and practice

■ promote the codes of practice to social care workers, service users and carers and cooperate with the Social Care Council's proceedings.

The codes of practice say that social care workers must:

■ protect the rights and promote the interests of service users and carers

■ make every effort to establish and maintain the trust and confidence of service users and carers

■ promote service users' independence whilst protecting them, as far as possible, from danger or harm

■ respect service users' rights whilst making sure that their behaviour doesn't harm themselves or others

■ maintain public trust and confidence in social care services

■ be accountable for the quality of their work and take responsibility for maintaining and improving their knowledge and skills.

You can read the codes of practice in full by visiting www.gscc.org.uk, www.ccwales.org.uk, www.niscc.info and www.sssc.uk.com.

Many health and social care providers have their own organisational codes of practice, which are specific to the service user group they work with. And many produce charters that describe how they aim to protect service users' rights and what people can do if they feel that their rights are being denied.

Links to Unit 3, page 70.

Responsibilities in protecting the rights of service users

Employers in health and social care settings have a responsibility to protect service users' rights.

Figure 4.9

Employers' responsibilities in protecting service users' rights

> By only employing staff who they have checked are suitable to work with vulnerable adults and children

> By writing policies and procedures that are based on the conventions, laws and regulations that protect human rights

How employers protect service users' rights

> By providing training and supervision that enable staff to understand their roles and responsibilities in protecting service users' rights

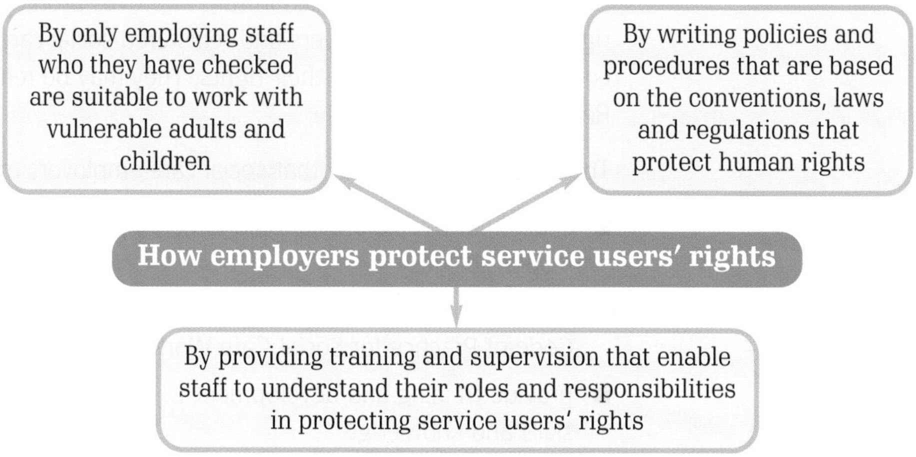

Health and social care workers have a responsibility to protect service users' rights by using the care values in their work. You read about the care values in Unit 1.

Links to Unit 1, pages 23–4.

Other ways in which health and care workers protect service users' rights include:

■ following codes of practice and workplace procedures

■ acting as an advocate for people who don't know their rights, lack the confidence to speak up for themselves and are confused

■ empowering people to exercise their rights, for example, by helping them find out what their rights are

■ challenging colleagues and service users if their behaviour appears to deny others their rights, even if it is unintended and accidental

■ reporting any concerns about denial of rights to their supervisor or manager

■ reflecting on how well they protect service users' rights. They should also ask for feedback about their work practice from the people they work with, and act on feedback if it will improve their work practice.

remember

Despite our differences, we all have the same rights. In addition, we all have a responsibility to protect other people's rights. Health and care workers have a special responsibility to protect the rights of service users.

Citizens Advice Bureau www.citizensadvice.org.uk

Figure 4.10
Bridge Street Luncheon Club

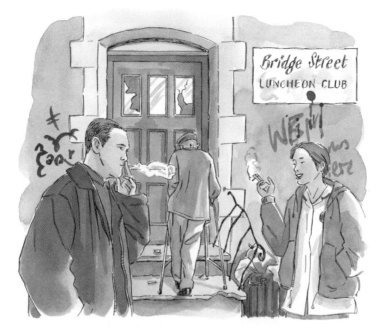

case study 4.4

Promoting rights

Bridge Street Luncheon Club provides a social outlet for a diverse range of local people who either live on their own or who are unable to prepare their own meals. The kitchen staff have limited cooking experience and the meals they prepare and serve are the same, day after day after day...

Not one of the staff working at Bridge Street has received or is interested in having any training. As a result, many don't understand their job role. Some have no experience of working with people and have a negative attitude to their work. For example, they are discourteous and impatient and not always clean and appropriately dressed. And they treat all the service users in the same way, regardless of any differences.

The employer, who also manages Bridge Street, rarely emerges from her office, where she keeps personal information about staff and service users. She won't let anyone else go into the office because the records she keeps are confidential.

Locks on the toilet doors are broken, there is no running hot water and the steps up into the building are cracked and uneven. There are no security systems in place and anyone is free to come and go in the building.

There is a growing feeling of discontent with the way that the luncheon club is run but many of the service users find it difficult to speak up. This is because they lack confidence or have problems making themselves understood. Neither the staff nor the manager have the time or compassion to find out how they feel.

activity

GROUP WORK

(a) List the service users' rights which are not being protected at the luncheon club.

(b) How would getting to understand service users as individuals help the staff and manager to promote their rights?

(c) What laws and codes of practice are not being upheld by the staff and manager at the club?

(d) Explain how not upholding these laws and codes of practice fails to support service users' rights.

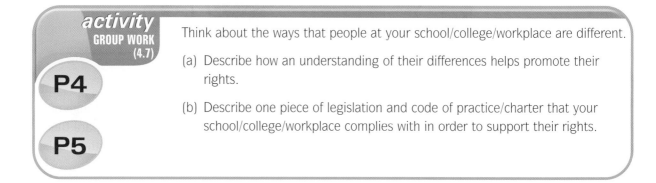

activity

GROUP WORK
(4.7)

P4

P5

Think about the ways that people at your school/college/workplace are different.

(a) Describe how an understanding of their differences helps promote their rights.

(b) Describe one piece of legislation and code of practice/charter that your school/college/workplace complies with in order to support their rights.

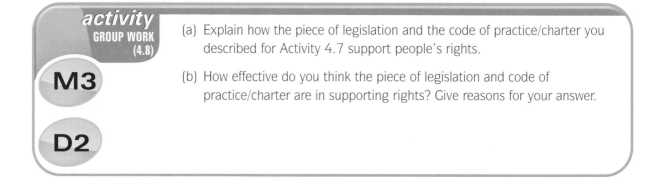

activity

GROUP WORK
(4.8)

M3

D2

(a) Explain how the piece of legislation and the code of practice/charter you described for Activity 4.7 support people's rights.

(b) How effective do you think the piece of legislation and code of practice/charter are in supporting rights? Give reasons for your answer.

*progress
check*

1. Describe five social and political factors that make us different from each other.

2. Compare the practices and beliefs of people from two different religious or secular beliefs.

3. Describe three factors that can affect people's access to equal opportunity.

4. Explain, using examples, why health and social care services need to be different in order to promote equal opportunities for service users.

5. Give three examples of discriminatory practice experienced by service users.

6. Describe three ways in which health and social care workers can overcome discriminatory practice.

7. Explain how discrimination can affect people physically, intellectually, emotionally and socially.

8. Name five basic human rights.

9. Describe how the rights of service users are protected.

10. Describe how understanding diversity can help health and social care workers promote the rights of service users.

Books

Gresford, P. (1997), *Case Studies in Health and Social Care* (Heinemann)

Meggitt, C. (1997), *A Special Needs Handbook for Health and Social Care* (Hodder Arnold)

Michie, V. (2004), *Working in Care Settings* (Nelson Thornes)

Moonie, N., Bates, A. and Spencer-Perkins, D. (2004), *Diversity and Rights in Care* (*Care Management Series*) (Heinemann)

O'Hagan, K. (2001), *Cultural Competence in the Caring Professions* (Jessica Kingsley)

Skelt, A. (1993), *Caring for People with Disabilities* (Pearson)

Social Exclusion Unit (2005), *Improving Services. Improving Lives* (ODPM)

Windsor, G. and Moonie, N. (eds) (2000), *GNVQ Health and Social Care: Intermediate Compulsory Units with Edexcel Options* (Heinemann)

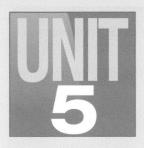

Anatomy and Physiology for Health and Social Care

This unit covers:

- the organisation of the human body
- the structure, function and interrelationship of major body systems
- how monitoring body systems through routine measurements and observations can indicate malfunction
- malfunctions in body systems and the resultant needs of service users.

In order to promote and maintain service users' health and well-being, health and social care workers need to have a knowledge and understanding of the anatomy and physiology of the body, how to monitor the way the body works and the reasons for making measurements and observations. They need to understand the importance of accuracy and of following health and safety procedures when making measurements and observations. They also need to understand how and why the body may malfunction and the care that service users need in the event of ill health.

grading criteria

To achieve a **Pass** grade the evidence must show that the learner is able to:	To achieve a **Merit** grade the evidence must show that the learner is able to:	To achieve a **Distinction** grade the evidence must show that the learner is able to:
P1 identify the position and function/s of the main organs of the human body Pg 110	**M1** explain the structure of two body systems in relation to their functions Pg 114	**D1** explain how two systems of the body interrelate to perform a named function Pg 116
P2 describe the structure and functions of two of the major body systems Pg 114	**M2** explain how routine measurements and observations taken on these two body systems could indicate malfunction Pg 122	**D2** explain how routine measurements and observations can be used as indicators of health/ill health Pg 125
P3 describe the routine measurements and observations used to monitor these two body systems Pg 122		

grading criteria

To achieve a **Pass** grade the evidence must show that the learner is able to:	To achieve a **Merit** grade the evidence must show that the learner is able to:	To achieve a **Distinction** grade the evidence must show that the learner is able to:
P4 identify a malfunction in each of the two major body systems described　Pg 126	**M3** explain the link between the malfunction of the two body systems and the care the patients/service users receive　Pg 126	
P5 identify risk factors for each of the two malfunctions　Pg 126		
P6 describe the care that should be given to patients/service users with these two malfunctions　Pg 126		

The Organisation of the Human Body

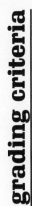

Anatomy
keyword
The structure of the body, i.e. the way different parts of the body are put together.

The first stage in understanding the **anatomy** and **physiology** of the body is to consider its basic organisation.

Organisation

The body is organised into cells, tissues, organs and systems.

www.bbc.co.uk/science
www.bupa.co.uk/health_information

Cells

Cells are the **microscopic** building blocks from which all living things are made. They have the same basic parts:

- a nucleus, which is the 'brain' of the cell and controls how it works
- cytoplasm, which is a jelly-like fluid containing the organelles that enable the cell to work
- a cell membrane, which surrounds and protects the cell.

Physiology
keyword
The function of the body, i.e. the way different parts of the body work, both on their own and together.

Microscopic
keyword
Very, very small. Anything that is microscopic can only be seen through the lens of a microscope.

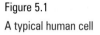
Figure 5.1

A typical human cell

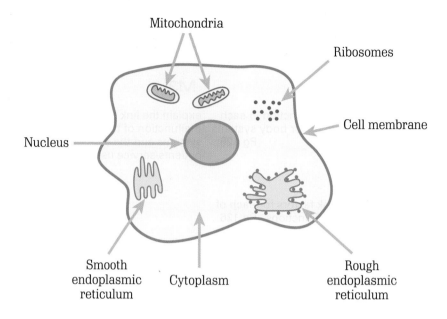

There are many types of cell in the human body, each having a different function.

Figure 5.2

Cells in the human body

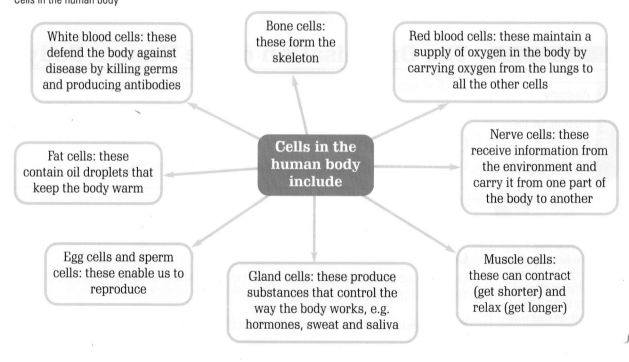

White blood cells: these defend the body against disease by killing germs and producing antibodies

Bone cells: these form the skeleton

Red blood cells: these maintain a supply of oxygen in the body by carrying oxygen from the lungs to all the other cells

Fat cells: these contain oil droplets that keep the body warm

Cells in the human body include

Nerve cells: these receive information from the environment and carry it from one part of the body to another

Egg cells and sperm cells: these enable us to reproduce

Gland cells: these produce substances that control the way the body works, e.g. hormones, sweat and saliva

Muscle cells: these can contract (get shorter) and relax (get longer)

Tissues

A tissue is composed of cells that have the same function. For example, blood tissue is composed of blood cells and bone tissue of bone cells. The cells within a tissue are held together by a matrix that allows movement of substances in and out of the cells. In blood tissue this matrix is a fluid called plasma and in bone tissue it is a hard material containing calcium.

Organs

An organ is a part of the body that is made up from more than one type of tissue. This means that an organ has more than one function. The main organs in the human body are the skin, heart, lungs, brain, eyes, ears, stomach, pancreas, intestines, liver, kidneys, bladder, ovaries (female), testes (male) and uterus (female).

Location of the organs in the body

Figure 5.3

Location of organs in the body

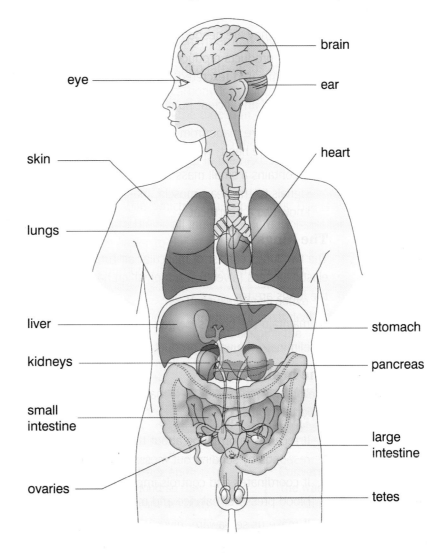

- brain
- eye
- ear
- skin
- heart
- lungs
- liver
- stomach
- kidneys
- pancreas
- small intestine
- large intestine
- ovaries
- tetes

The main functions of organs
The skin

The skin is the largest organ in the body. It contains a number of different tissues so has a variety of functions:

- It surrounds and protects the body.
- It helps maintain body temperature.

The kidneys

The function of the kidneys is to purify the blood. As blood passes through the kidneys, excess salt and water, and waste products such as urea, are filtered out to make urine, which is passed to the bladder.

The bladder

The function of the bladder is to store urine until it is eliminated from the body. The opening through which urine passes is controlled by a ring of muscle. When the pressure of urine in the bladder reaches a certain level, the muscle relaxes and the bladder walls contract, forcing urine to flow from the body. Urinary continence is the ability to control this flow of urine.

The testes and ovaries

The function of the testes is to produce and store sperm cells and that of the ovaries is to produce and store egg cells. Fusion of a human egg and sperm cell creates a baby, in a process known as reproduction. The testes and ovaries also produce hormones, which you will read about in the next section.

The uterus

The muscular uterus also plays a role in reproduction. Its functions are to:

- protect and feed an unborn baby as it develops
- contract and push the baby down the birth canal when it is ready to be born.

keyword

Body system
A group of organs working together to carry out one or more functions.

---

link

Links to Unit 6, page 130.

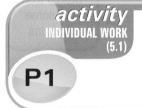

activity
INDIVIDUAL WORK (5.1)

P1

Draw a labelled diagram of the human body to show the location of the skin, heart, lungs, brain, eyes, ears, stomach, pancreas, intestines, liver, kidneys, bladder, ovaries, testes and uterus, and describe the main function of each organ.

The Structure, Function and Inter-relationship of Major Body Systems

The previous section described the structure and function of some important cells, tissues and organs. This section introduces you to the structure and function of some major **body systems** and how they work together.

www.bbc.co.uk/science
www.bupa.co.uk/health_information

The structure and function of body systems
The cardiovascular system

The cardiovascular system comprises:

- the heart
- blood vessels
- blood.

Its functions are to maintain the body's supply of oxygen and to transport materials around the body.

You read earlier that the heart pumps blood around the body under pressure. Circulation of the blood ensures that all body cells have a supply of oxygen and that nutrients (digested food), hormones and antibodies are transported to the parts of the body where they are needed. The circulation also ensures that waste products, such as carbon dioxide and urea, are transported away from body cells to where they can be eliminated.

Blood circulates around the body in blood vessels. The table below describes the three different types of blood vessel.

Table 5.1 Blood vessels

Type of vessel	Direction of blood flow	Blood pressure within the vessel	Features
Artery	Away from the heart to all the body cells	High: when an artery is cut, blood spurts out under pressure.	Artery walls are thick and very elastic. The blood they carry (except in the pulmonary artery) is bright red due to high oxygen content.
Capillary	From the arteries to the veins, between the cells	Medium	Capillary walls are very thin, allowing oxygen and nutrients to pass out into the cells and cell waste products to pass into the capillary.
Vein	From the body cells back to the heart	Low: when a vein is cut, blood only oozes out.	Vein walls are thin and not very elastic. The blood they carry (except in the pulmonary vein) is dark red due to low oxygen content.

The respiratory system

The respiratory system comprises:

- the nose, through which oxygen-rich air is inhaled and carbon dioxide-rich air is exhaled (breathing)
- the larynx, trachea and bronchi, which are the air tubes that connect the nose with the lungs
- the lungs, which are made up of bronchioles and alveoli
- blood vessels, which circulate around the alveoli
- the muscles of the chest cavity.

The respiratory system has two main functions: to maintain the body's supply of oxygen and to eliminate the waste product carbon dioxide.

When the chest muscles contract, the chest cavity increases and air is sucked into the lungs (inhalation). Blood circulating around the alveoli absorbs oxygen from the inhaled air and is pumped around the body, maintaining the body's oxygen supply. At the same time, carbon dioxide passes from the blood into the alveoli. When the chest muscles relax, the chest cavity decreases and carbon dioxide is pushed out of the lungs (exhalation). This is how the lungs eliminate the waste product carbon dioxide.

The nervous system

The main function of the nervous system is to receive information about the environment so that the body can respond appropriately.

The nervous system comprises:

- the brain and spinal cord (the central nervous system – CNS)
- sense organs, which receive information about the environment:
  - outside the body, i.e. the skin, eyes, ears, nose and tongue; they sense touch, pressure, pain, heat, cold, light, sound, smell and taste
  - inside the body; they are in the ears, muscles and organs and sense, for example, the body's position and heartbeat
- sensory nerves, which carry information from the sense organs to the CNS
- relay nerves, which are in the CNS and form a link between sensory and motor nerves
- motor nerves, which carry information from the CNS to effectors
- effectors (muscles and glands), which respond to information coming from the CNS. When a muscle receives information, it contracts; when a gland receives information, it produces a secretion, e.g. a hormone, sweat, saliva.

For example, if you touch a very hot object, sensory nerves in your skin would carry information about the heat to your brain. Your brain would respond by sending a message along motor nerves to the muscles in your hand. As a result, the muscles would contract, moving your hand away from the heat and preventing you from getting burned.

The nervous system also coordinates and controls our skeletal muscles (the muscles connected to our bones) so that we move smoothly and stay balanced.

The endocrine system

The endocrine system consists of a number of different glands. Its function is to produce hormones which coordinate and control the way the body works.

The digestive system

The function of the digestive system is the digestion of food materials. You read about the organs and enzymes that are involved in digestion in the previous section.

Table 5.2 Structure and function of the endocrine system

Endocrine gland	Location	Hormones produced	Function of the hormones
Pituitary gland	Just below the brain	A range of hormones	Control other endocrine glands
Adrenal glands	Above the kidneys	Adrenaline and corticosteroids	Adrenaline prepares the body for action; corticosteroids control blood pressure and the level of chemicals in the body
Thyroid gland	In front of the larynx	Thyroid hormone	Controls the speed at which cells work (metabolic rate)
Parathyroid gland	Behind the thyroid	Parathyroid hormone	Controls the amount of calcium in the blood
Pancreas	Behind the stomach	Insulin and glucagon	Insulin reduces and glucagon increases the blood glucose level
Testes (male)	In the scrotum that hangs below the abdomen	Androgens	Control the development and functioning of the male sex organs and the development of male secondary sexual characteristics (muscles, broadening of the shoulders, growth of body and facial hair)
Ovaries (female)	In the lower abdomen	Oestrogen and progesterone	Oestrogen controls the development and functioning of the female sex organs and the development of female secondary sexual characteristics (breasts, broadening of the hips, growth of body hair, menstruation); progesterone prepares the body for and maintains pregnancy

The excretory system

The function of the excretory system is the excretion or elimination of waste products from the body. The organs that make up the excretory system are:

- the skin, which eliminates water, salt and urea in sweat
- the lungs, which eliminate carbon dioxide in expired air
- the kidneys, which eliminate water, salt, urea, hormones, alcohol and drugs in urine.

You read about the skin, lungs and kidneys in the previous section.

The reproductive system

The male reproductive system comprises:

- two testicles, which produce and store sperm cells and produce male hormones
- sperm tubes, which carry sperm away from the testicles to the penis
- a prostate gland and a seminal vesicle, which produce a fluid that mixes with sperm to form semen

- insulin, which reduces blood glucose level by making the liver and muscles take glucose from the blood and store it as glycogen
- glucagon, which increases blood glucose level by making the liver break glycogen down and release glucose back into the blood.

Maintenance of blood pressure

Blood pressure (BP) is the force that makes blood flow from the heart, through the arteries, capillaries and veins, and back to the heart. BP has to stay within narrow limits.

There are a number of body systems and organs that act together to control blood pressure, including:

- the nervous system, which responds to a drop in blood pressure by constricting blood vessels and increasing the force with which blood leaves the heart
- the endocrine system, which changes blood pressure by dilating or constricting blood vessels and increasing the amount of blood pumped out by the heart
- the kidneys, which respond to changes in blood pressure by increasing or decreasing the volume and concentration of circulating blood.

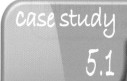

case study

5.1

The London Marathon

John has entered the London Marathon dressed as a heart for a local charity. It is a very hot day, there is no opportunity to eat and John is nervous about his performance. He wants to win!

activity
INDIVIDUAL WORK

(a) How will the event affect John's body temperature, blood glucose level and blood pressure?

(b) How will his body temperature, blood glucose level and blood pressure be maintained?

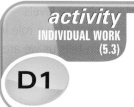

activity
INDIVIDUAL WORK
(5.3)

D1

Explain in your own words how two body systems work together to maintain the body in good health.

How Monitoring Body Systems through Routine Measurements and Observations can Indicate Malfunction

You read above that good health is dependent on conditions within our bodies staying within narrow limits. There are limits for all physiological processes, as there are normal signs of good health. Measurements and observations that don't fall within a normal range signify ill health. This is the reason why health and care workers need to be able to make routine measurements and observations.

www.bbc.co.uk
www.nhsdirect.nhs.uk
www.netdoctor.co.uk

keyword

Sharps
Hazardous sharp equipment such as needles, scalpel blades, scissors, razors and lancets.

Health and safety

Some measurements and observations are simple and straightforward. Others involve contact with hazardous substances such as glass, **sharps** and body fluids. Health and care workers have a responsibility to reduce risks to health and safety by:

- only making measurements in which they have been trained and are competent

- following workplace procedures and manufacturers' instructions to ensure they use equipment correctly

- following workplace procedures when disposing of used equipment and hazardous substances to prevent accidents and control the spread of infection.

Safe working practices promote service users' rights to be protected from danger and harm and ensure that workers comply with the health and safety legislation you read about in Unit 2 (HASWA 1974, COSHH 1994, MHSWR 1999).

Links to Unit 2, pages 47–51.

Some of the routine measurements and observations made in health and social care settings are described below. Note that when in doubt, even a competent worker should double check their measurements and observations by repeating the measurement or asking a colleague for a second opinion. Accuracy is of vital importance as it can mean the difference between life and death.

Routine physiological measurements
Body temperature

The expected range of body temperature is 36.5°C–37.2°C (97.7°F–99°F). Body temperature can be measured using:

- a thermometer, placed in the mouth or armpit. Measurements made in the armpit are about 0.5 °C lower than the body's core temperature so 0.5 °C must be added or an inaccurate measurement will be recorded. And if a person has just eaten something hot or cold, a thermometer in the mouth will also give an inaccurate measurement.

- thermometer strips, which are placed on the forehead and give approximate measurements such as whether the person is too hot or too cold. They are quick and easy to use but not as accurate as a thermometer.

- an ear thermometer, which is very accurate and quick to use. If the person has been lying on a warm pillow or out in the cold, wait about 15 minutes for his or her temperature to adjust or you will record an inaccurate measurement.

Pulse rate

The pulse is a wave of pressure that passes along the arteries and is caused by the pumping of the heart. It can be felt where an artery is close to the skin and can be pressed against a bone, e.g. the radial pulse in the wrist. When feeling for the radial pulse, place your three middle fingertips on the inside wrist in line with the base of the thumb and press lightly against the bone.

The pulse rate is the number of pulses per minute and is the rate at which the heart beats. The expected range for an adult is between 60 and 100 beats per minute. When taking someone's pulse rate, don't use your thumb as it has its own pulse and will give you an inaccurate measurement!

Blood pressure (BP)

You read earlier that BP is the force that makes blood flow from the heart around the body and back to the heart. It is usually measured using an electronic device: human error when using the traditional sphygmomanometer is likely to give an inaccurate measurement.

BP increases with age and body weight but the expected range for an adult is between '90 over 60' and '120 over 80' (90/60 mmHg–120/80 mmHg).

- The first number is the systolic blood pressure – the maximum pressure in the arteries when the heart contracts and pushes blood out into the body.

- The second number is the diastolic blood pressure – the minimum pressure in the arteries when the heart relaxes and fills with blood.

Figure 5.7

Taking a pulse

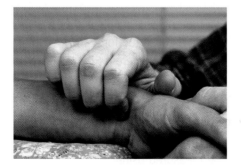

Breathing rate

Breathing rate is the number of breaths taken per minute and the expected range for an adult is 16–18 per minute. Breathing rate can be measured by:

■ watching or pressing lightly on a person's chest and counting the number of times the chest rises and falls

■ putting your face close to their mouth and nose and counting the number of breaths you feel on your cheek.

Both methods require concentration to prevent inaccurate measurements.

Blood glucose levels

The blood glucose level is the amount of glucose in the blood. The expected range of blood glucose levels is 4–8mmol/litre.

Blood glucose level can be measured using a blood glucose level testing kit, which contains a number of strips and a measuring device.

1. Place the strip into the device.

2. Take a blood sample by pricking the person's finger with a sharp lancet.

3. Put a drop of blood on the strip.

4. Wait for the device to display the blood glucose level.

Peak flow

Peak flow is the measure of how fast air can be blown out of the lungs, which in turn gives a measure of the width of the airways. Peak flow readings vary according to age, sex and height and are often lower in the morning than in the evening. The expected range of peak flow readings is published on a chart, to which health and care workers must refer when making measurements.

Figure 5.8

Measuring breathing rate

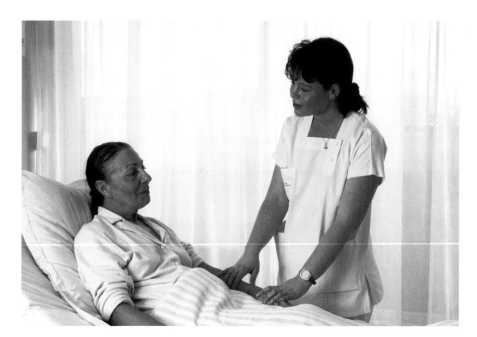

Peak flow is measured using a peak flow meter.

1. Put the marker to zero.
2. Ask the person to take a deep breath in and seal his or her lips around the mouthpiece.
3. Ask the person to blow as hard and as fast as possible into the meter.
4. Note the reading.

Repeat twice, to give three readings, and record the best of the three. It is important to do this correctly. Not blowing hard enough and a poor seal between lips and mouthpiece will give inaccurate measurements.

Figure 5.9
Measuring peak flow

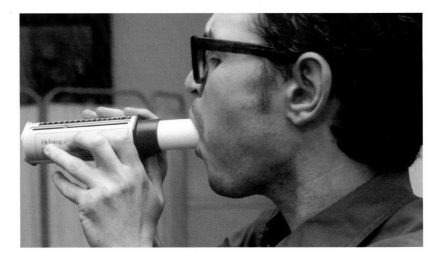

Routine observations
Abnormal breathing rates and rhythms

You read above that the expected breathing rate for an adult is 16–18 breaths per minute. Service users' breathing should be observed and any:

- breathlessness and changes in the depth, rhythm and sound of breathing, e.g. wheezing
- tenderness and pain whilst breathing

should be reported to an appropriate person without delay.

Skin colour and texture

Healthy young skin glows, regardless of a person's racial background. It is firm, smooth, possibly freckled and has an even tone. As skin ages, it loses its elasticity and becomes lined and wrinkled. It may become coarse and mottled, and develop age spots and enlarged pores.

Service users' skin colour and tone should be observed and any changes reported to an appropriate person without delay. Characteristics that can indicate ill health include:

Figure 5.10

Making a routine observation

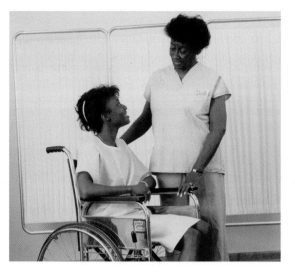

- changes in colour, e.g. flushing, pallor, blueness (cyanosis), purpleness
- fluid retention or puffiness (oedema)
- a dry, clammy, sweaty or unusually hot or cold surface
- spots, rashes, blisters, open sores and changes in the appearance of moles
- tenderness and pain.

Coughing and the expulsion of sputum

Coughing is a natural reaction that occurs when 'things go down the wrong way' and when there is excess mucus in the airways. Service users' coughing and sputum should be observed and any:

- unusual episodes of coughing, e.g. choking
- unusual noises or vomiting
- changes in the amount and appearance of sputum and mucus, e.g. colour, thickness, presence of blood

should be reported to an appropriate person without delay.

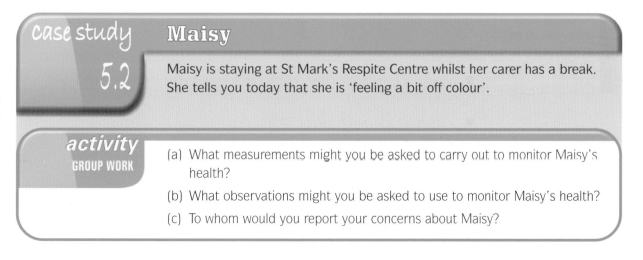

case study 5.2 — Maisy

Maisy is staying at St Mark's Respite Centre whilst her carer has a break. She tells you today that she is 'feeling a bit off colour'.

activity
GROUP WORK

(a) What measurements might you be asked to carry out to monitor Maisy's health?

(b) What observations might you be asked to use to monitor Maisy's health?

(c) To whom would you report your concerns about Maisy?

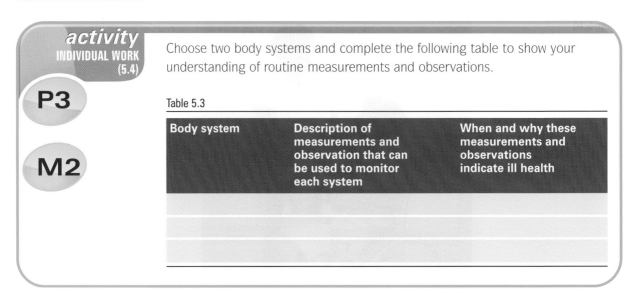

activity
INDIVIDUAL WORK
(5.4)

P3

M2

Choose two body systems and complete the following table to show your understanding of routine measurements and observations.

Table 5.3

Body system	Description of measurements and observation that can be used to monitor each system	When and why these measurements and observations indicate ill health

Malfunctions in Body Systems and the Resultant Needs of Service Users

Ill health occurs when body systems malfunction. This section looks at a number of ill health conditions, the risk factors that are associated with them and the care needs of service users experiencing the conditions.

www.nhsdirect.nhs.uk
www.bbc.co.uk/health

Malfunctions and risk factors
Coronary heart disease (CHD)

CHD is a disease of the cardiovascular system. It occurs when arteries taking blood to the heart walls become furred up with **atheroma** and are unable to maintain a supply of oxygen to the heart. Symptoms include breathlessness, oedema, cyanosis, weakness, nausea and sweating.

CHD can cause:

- angina, a pain in the chest, which can spread to the shoulders, neck and arms

- a heart attack, which can be fatal.

Risk factors that increase the likelihood of CHD include:

- **age**. The risk of developing CHD increases with age.

- **gender**. Before the menopause, women have a lower risk of developing CHD than men.

keyword

Atheroma
A thick, fatty sludge which forms plaques on artery walls, reducing the space through which blood can flow.

■ **inherited factors**. A family history of CHD increases the risk of it developing.

■ **lifestyle factors** such as smoking, lack of exercise and a fatty diet.

Links to Unit 9, page 205.

Stroke

A stroke results from a malfunction of the cardiovascular system. It is caused by burst blood vessels or blood clots in the brain, which starve the brain of oxygen, damaging or killing cells. People who have had a stroke are often left with communication and mobility difficulties.

Risk factors that increase the likelihood of a stroke include:

■ **age**. The risk of having a stroke increases with age.

■ **lifestyle factors** such as unhealthy eating, smoking and alcohol abuse.

Figure 5.11

Malfunctioning body systems: diabetes, chronic bronchitis and asthma

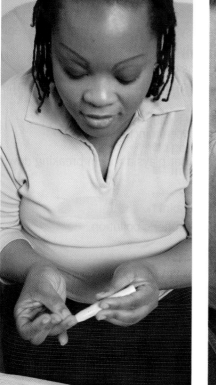
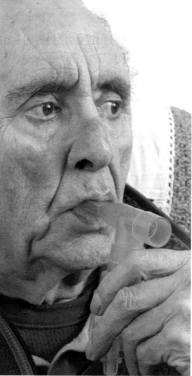
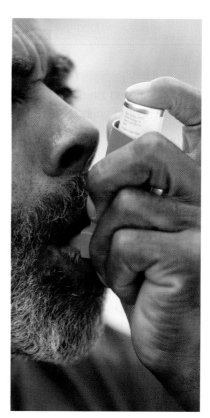

Asthma

Asthma is a disease of the pulmonary system. It is caused by inflamed and constricted airways and an excess production of mucus. When someone has an asthma attack, their chest becomes tight, they wheeze, cough and have difficulty breathing.

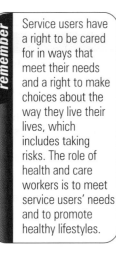 **remember**
Service users have a right to be cared for in ways that meet their needs and a right to make choices about the way they live their lives, which includes taking risks. The role of health and care workers is to meet service users' needs and to promote healthy lifestyles.

- carefully monitoring their condition and reporting any changes to an appropriate person without delay
- keeping them warm and comfortable and making sure that pressure ulcers don't develop in people who are chair or bed bound
- actively supporting them to take their medication, eat a healthy diet, stop smoking, etc.
- encouraging them to do as much as they can for themselves, to maintain their independence and physical ability
- following health and safety and infection control procedures at all times.

 link

Links to Unit 2, pages 29–32.

---

activity
INDIVIDUAL WORK
(5.6)

P4

P5

Find out about two diseases and produce a poster for each that shows:

(a) the body systems that are malfunctioning

(b) the risk factors associated with each disease.

---

activity
INDIVIDUAL WORK
(5.7)

P6

M3

Write an information sheet for care workers that:

(a) describes a disease commonly experienced by a service user group of your choice

(b) identifies the body systems that are malfunctioning

(c) describes the care that needs to be given to service users who experience these diseases

(d) explains why this care needs to be given.

progress check

1   Name five body organs and describe their location in the body.

2. Name five body systems and explain the link between their structure and function.

3   List the ill health conditions that can occur in each of these five systems.

4. Identify the risk factors for each of these ill health conditions.

5. Describe three routine measurements and three routine observations made in health and social care settings.

6. Describe measurements and observations that would indicate the ill health conditions you listed for question 3.

7. How would you care for service users experiencing these ill health conditions?

Books

Mackean, D. G. (1988), *Human Life* (John Murray)

Mackean, D. G. and Jones, B. (1987), *Introduction to Human and Social Biology* (John Murray)

Minett, P., Wayne, D. and Rubenstein, D. (1999), *Health Sciences* (Collins Educational)

Page, M. (ed) (2005), *The Human Body* (Dorling Kindersley)

Windsor, G. and Moonie, N. (ed) (2000), GNVQ *Health and Social Care: Intermediate Compulsory Units with Edexcel Options* (Heinemann)

Wright, D. (2000), *Human Physiology and Health* (Heinemann)

Wright, D. (2001), *Human Physiology and Health for GCSE: Resource Pack* (Heinemann)

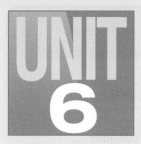

UNIT 6

Human Lifespan Development

This unit covers:

- the developmental changes that occur at different life stages
- the positive and negative influences on individuals at different life stages
- the factors that can influence an individual's self-concept
- the changing care needs at different life stages.

To enable them to meet care needs effectively at different stages in service users' lives, health and social care workers need to know and understand the key aspects of and influences on human growth and development. This unit aims to help people who want to work in health and social care develop their understanding of physical, intellectual, emotional and social growth and development, the positive and negative influences on growth and development and the changing care needs of individuals at different life stages.

grading criteria

To achieve a **Pass** grade the evidence must show that the learner is able to:	To achieve a **Merit** grade the evidence must show that the learner is able to:	To achieve a **Distinction** grade the evidence must show that the learner is able to:
P1 identify the key aspects of physical, intellectual, emotional and social development that takes place through the life stages Pg 133	**M1** describe the key aspects of physical, intellectual, emotional and social development that takes place through the life stages Pg 133	**D1** explain how growth and development at each life stage can be influenced positively and negatively Pg 139
P2 identify the positive and negative influences on growth and development Pg 139	**M2** explain how life events can affect the development and care needs of individuals Pg 148	**D2** explain how meeting individual care needs can improve the individual's self-concept Pg 146
P3 identify factors that influence the individual's self-concept Pg 143	**M3** describe how five different factors can influence the development of the individual's self-concept Pg 143	
P4 explain potential differences in the care needs of individuals at different life stages Pg 143		

The Developmental Changes that Occur at Different Life Stages

Life stages

There are seven main life stages during which people **grow** and **develop** physically, intellectually, emotionally and socially:

1. conception
2. birth and infancy (0–3 years)
3. childhood (4–10 years)
4. adolescence (11–18 years)
5. adulthood (19–65 years)
6. old age (65+ years)
7. the final stages of life, preparing for death.

keyword

Grow
Become bigger, in size or in number.

keyword

Develop
Become more complex.

Figure 6.1

Different life stages

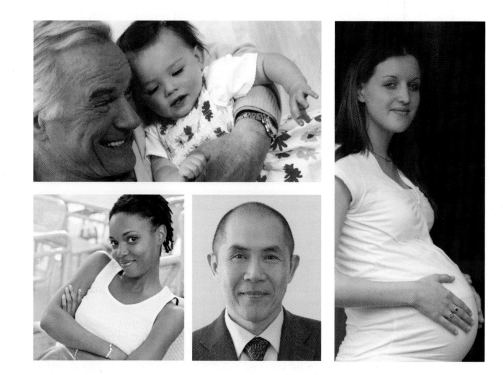

Key aspects of development
Physical growth and development

Physical growth and development is to do with changes in body size and complexity.

Table 6.1 Key aspects of physical growth and development

Life stage	Key aspects of physical growth and development
Conception	Growth begins at conception, when a sperm cell fertilises an egg cell. In the first three months of pregnancy the fertilised egg cell divides to produce cells which grow and develop into the tissues and organs of the foetus. The foetus continues to grow until it is mature enough to be born at about nine months.
Infancy and childhood	Infants and children grow rapidly. They also develop sensory skills (sight, hearing, smell and taste); manipulative skills (using the hands); hand–eye coordination (using sight and manipulative skills together); and motor skills (crawling, walking, running).
Adolescence	Puberty, which occurs during adolescence, marks the change from childhood to adulthood. It is when the reproductive organs grow and mature, secondary sexual characteristics develop, and bones and muscles grow, giving the body shape and strength.
Adulthood	The main function of growth in adulthood is to repair and replace worn out cells and tissues. Menopause, which occurs in women in late adulthood, is when hormonal changes cause a reduction of calcium in the bones. As a result, post-menopausal women can lose height and are at risk of osteoporosis (weak, brittle bones).
Old age	In the ageing body, cell and tissue repair slows down, which is why older people often experience weight loss; the bones lose calcium, become brittle and the person loses height; the muscles lose their strength; and the sense organs become less efficient, resulting in loss of sight, hearing, smell and taste.

Intellectual development

Intellectual development is to do with the development of communication and language, learning, understanding, thinking and problem-solving skills, and memory. Intellectual development carries on throughout life – you're never too old to learn!

Table 6.2 Key aspects of intellectual development

Life stage	Key aspects of intellectual development
Birth and infancy	From the moment of birth, infants communicate their needs by crying. At about three months they can communicate with their carer by showing recognition and smiling. At about six months they are able to communicate different needs in different ways. At about nine months they can say and understand a few simple words. From about twelve months their language skills and understanding increase rapidly until at about four years they can hold simple conversations, ask questions and understand, remember and tell favourite stories and nursery rhymes.
Childhood	There is rapid learning in childhood. Children develop thinking skills, an understanding of numbers, and language skills as they learn to read and write. They start to develop a self-concept (you will learn about self-concept shortly) and to learn the difference between right and wrong (moral development). Moral behaviour is learnt through being rewarded or seeing other people rewarded for being good. Children learn not to behave badly if being naughty results in some sort of punishment.
Adolescence	In adolescence, young people start to think for themselves. They also develop the ability to think more deeply about things and to use their judgement to solve problems.
Adulthood	Intellectual development continues in adulthood, when people have to be able to make decisions and learn how to live independently, hold down a job, manage finances and be responsible for themselves and other people, etc.
Old age	Old age is not a reason to stop learning! However, the older people get, the longer it takes them to learn new things and the harder it is to remember recent events.

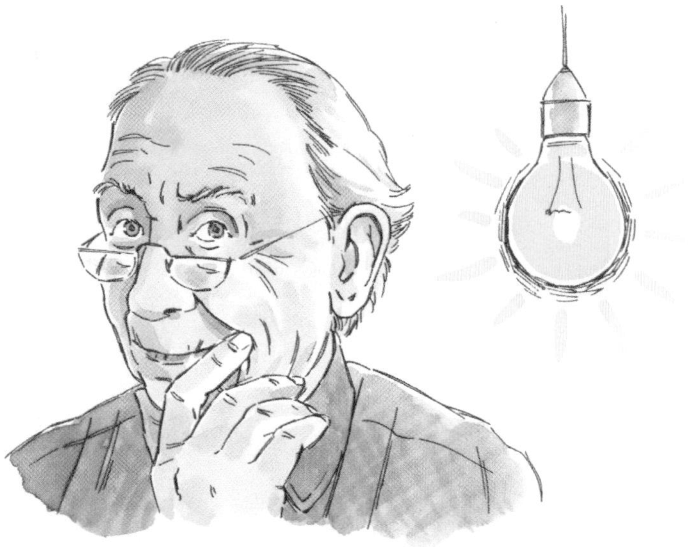

Figure 6.2
You're never too old to learn!

keyword
Peers
People in the same age group, social group, etc.

keyword
Empathetic
Being able to understand someone by 'putting yourself in their shoes'.

Emotional development

Emotional development is to do with the development of feelings, self-confidence and independence.

Table 6.3 Key aspects of emotional development

Life stage	Key aspects of emotional development
Infancy	'Bonding' is the word used to describe the process by which an emotional attachment is formed between an infant and a close carer. The bond develops as infant and carer communicate with each other through smiling, touching and making eye contact. Its purpose is to make sure the infant feels secure and to promote in the carer the need to protect the infant. Bonding takes about seven months, after which an infant often cries when left with a stranger. Infants become more affectionate with other people from about the age of one. By the age of two, they are very self-absorbed, demanding and quick-tempered. By three, they are more independent, less self-centred and are beginning to share.
Childhood	Children are able to share, play together and form friendships with each other. Older children begin to show signs of understanding and compassion for their **peers**.
Adolescence	Adolescence is a period of intense emotional change. The hormones which control puberty and sexual maturity can create confusion, loss of self-confidence, mood swings and changes in behaviour. Adolescents strive to be independent and friendships can become very intense.
Adulthood and old age	Adults and elderly people experience and learn to deal with a variety of positive and negative emotions, including the feelings associated with loss of independence due to ill health and old age. Having direct experience of a range of emotions enables people to be **empathetic** and wise.

Figure 6.3

Emotional and social development

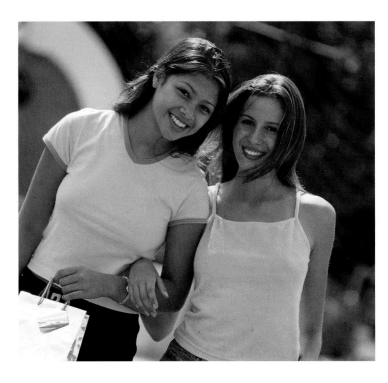

Social/cultural development

Social/cultural development is to do with developing relationships and beliefs and living and working with others.

Table 6.4 Key aspects of social development

Life stage	Key aspects of social development
Infancy	Infants form their first relationships with close family and people who provide them with a secure environment, such as early years care workers. Infancy is the time when social skills, such as being polite and having good manners, start to develop.
Childhood	When children start school, they develop new relationships, begin to understand their **social role** and start to learn the rules of behaviour outside the home. This helps them to interact with others in ways that involve cooperation and teamwork. They also start to learn **norms of behaviour** and the beliefs or values that underpin these norms.
Adolescence	Adolescence is a time for developing and learning from relationships, learning how to deal with **peer pressure** and developing personal beliefs, values and a **code of conduct**, which can conflict with those of their parents and authority.
Adulthood	Adults develop relationships with friends, partners, work colleagues and by starting their own family. Their social role continually develops and changes within the family, community and workplace.
Old age	Retirement and loss of friends, health and independence affect the ability of older people to make and maintain relationships. However, finding new things to do and taking part in activities helps them stay in touch with people and keep up their social role.

keyword

Social role
The part people play in their family, community, at school and work, etc.

keyword

Norms of behaviour
The way society expects us to behave in different situations.

keyword

Peer pressure
Pressure from one's peers to behave in a way that is similar to or acceptable by them.

keyword

Code of conduct
The standards which govern how people behave.

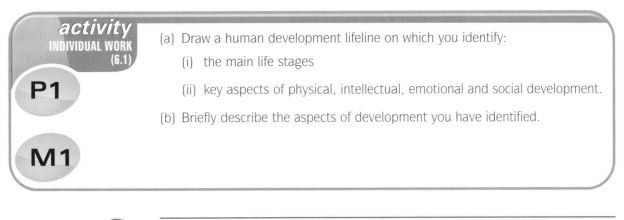

activity
INDIVIDUAL WORK
(6.1)

P1

M1

(a) Draw a human development lifeline on which you identify:

    (i) the main life stages

    (ii) key aspects of physical, intellectual, emotional and social development.

(b) Briefly describe the aspects of development you have identified.

The National Childbirth Trust www.nctpregnancyandbabycare.com

The Child Development Institute www.cdipage.com

www.zerotothree.org

The Pre-school Learning Alliance www.pre-school.org.uk

The British Association for Early Childhood Education www.early-education.org.uk

www.bbc.co.uk/parenting

www.ageconcern.org.uk

www.channel4.com/health

remember

Human growth and development continues throughout life with key changes occurring at different life stages.

The Positive and Negative Influences on Individuals at Different Life Stages

There are many factors that affect our growth and development and the following sections aim to improve your understanding of their positive and negative influences.

Socialisation

Socialisation is to do with teaching children to think and behave in ways that society and their family and culture expect of them. People who are not socialised find it difficult to make relationships and to belong to and be accepted by their culture and society.

Primary socialisation

Primary socialisation happens in a child's first few years and takes place in the home and family. It teaches the child family and cultural values, beliefs and behaviours, for example:

- to value members of their family, their home and the customs and traditions of the family's cultural background

- to believe in the religion of their family's choice

- to be polite, well mannered and behave according to the **role models** that the family exposes the child to.

keyword

Role model
Someone we copy because we respect and admire them.

The media

The media, for example newspapers, magazines, TV, film and radio, can have a negative effect on us throughout our lives. Its use of stereotypes, such as sexy young women and grumpy old men, can influence our ideas of how we and others should look and behave. And the way the media target men, women, boys or girls, for example sports coverage for males and beauty articles for females, can influence what we think we ought to know about and be interested in.

As you read in Unit 2, the media also have a positive influence. For example, TV documentaries, adverts and health promotion campaigns educate us, and much of what we see, hear and read in the media addresses everyday concerns, helping us to deal with relationship problems, financial worries, and so on.

 link

Links to Unit 2, page 38.

case study 6.2   Bert and Flo

Bert is 65 years old. He used to enjoy his job as a porter in a large hospital but the low wages meant that it was difficult to provide for his wife and children. He lives on his own in a council flat and occasionally meets up with a pal for a pint and to 'put the world right'. His children and grandchildren don't visit him as often as he would like.

Flo is also 65 years old. She used to be a teacher and has a good pension that allows her to live comfortably. She has no children but she has many nieces and nephews and a number of friends whom she meets frequently.

activity
GROUP WORK

Discuss the socio-economic factors that might have had an influence on Bert's and Flo's development.

Figure 6.5

Socio-economic factors that influence our development

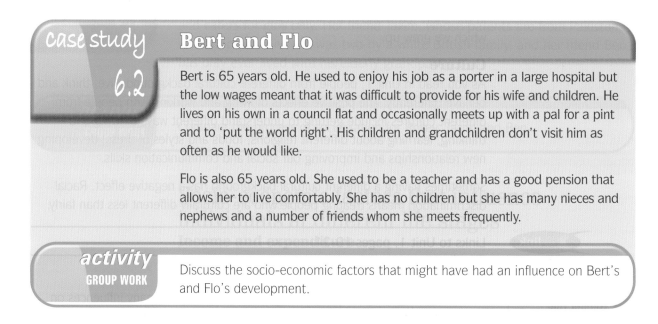

Links to Unit 4, page 91.

Life events that influence individuals at different life stages

Some life events are predictable, for example going to school, becoming a parent and bereavement. Others, like getting a divorce and becoming disabled, are unpredictable or unexpected. Whether we expect them or not, life events have an influence on our growth and development in the short, medium and long term, as the following examples demonstrate.

Birth of a sibling

The birth of a sibling (brother or sister) is usually a very happy occasion. It gives a child the opportunity to experience a different type of relationship, and to learn to share people and things and become sensible and responsible.

> **keyword**
>
> **Status**
> Position compared with others, e.g. sister, manager, chief inspector.

It can also be a traumatic occasion for a child. Their position in the family, for example as the only or youngest child, changes and they are treated and expected to behave in new ways. The child may feel 'pushed out', unloved, jealous and insecure. These feelings can stay with a person throughout their life. No doubt you are familiar with the feelings people have about their **status** in the family!

Going to nursery/school

Starting nursery or school can be exciting. However, unless a child is carefully prepared and supported, separation from their carer can be very stressful. A stressed child is at risk of being bullied, which can affect their ability to develop relationships for the rest of their life.

Nursery and school provide opportunities for development that have a positive influence throughout our lives. For example, we learn how to develop and maintain friendships and relationships with others; we develop language, communication and number skills, and we learn the importance of rules and cooperation and how to behave in new situations.

Moving house

Moving house gives us an opportunity to learn about a new area, develop a sense of belonging and a social role in a new community, meet new people and make new friends.

But pulling up our roots and establishing ourselves in a new neighbourhood can be unsettling. We don't all find it easy to make friends, be accepted by others and develop a sense of belonging. Unless we find a role to play in the new community, we may be lonely and socially isolated for as long as we live there.

Employment

Being offered a job gives us self-respect and respect from others. Doing the job allows us to learn and use new skills, grow in self-confidence, develop relationships with the people we work with, and, of course, become financially independent. With financial independence comes the opportunity to learn how to manage our earnings responsibly.

Leaving home

People leave home for a number of reasons, for example to get married or to go to a new job. Leaving home is a great leap forward for many people and helps build decision-making skills, self-confidence and independence. It also gives people a chance to develop their self-concept and social role and form new relationships.

Figure 6.6
Life events

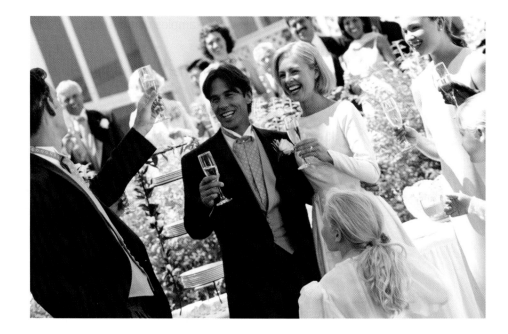

Marriage and parenthood

Marriage between two people who are in love is a joyous occasion and tells the world about their commitment to each other. People in loving, committed relationships nurture each others' self-confidence and self-esteem and learn to work as a team. They grow strong in the belief that someone loves them and that they can depend on each other.

Having a family is also very fulfilling. Parenthood involves a change in self-concept, an increase in social roles to include 'mother' or 'father', and becoming more responsible and less self-centred. It can change the relationship between partners and other family members but provides opportunities for developing new relationships with other parents.

Divorce

Divorce can be liberating! It can give people back their independence, help them build self-confidence and give them the chance to learn new skills and develop new relationships. Divorce can also be a long-term tragedy, destroying relationships, people's self-esteem and their trust in others.

Redundancy and retirement

Being made redundant or having to retire can also be liberating! At last there is time to do all the things you want to do, such as studying a course at college, rekindling relationships with old friends or doing some voluntary work.

However, for many people, losing their job means losing an important social role, status, self-confidence, self-esteem and income for the rest of their life. It also means losing the companionship of work colleagues, which can lead to loneliness, depression and the inability to develop new relationships.

Serious injury

Serious injury can cause physical disability and becoming disabled can change a person's life. Whilst many disabled people rise to the challenge that their disability presents, the effect of serious injury on others means they can find it difficult to maintain relationships, meet people and make new friends; they may have to change their job and living accommodation; and they may have to change their social role from 'carer' to 'cared for'. Changes like these can lead to a negative self-concept and to loss of self-confidence and independence.

Ageing and bereavement

The effects of growing old, which you read about earlier, can be emotionally and socially distressing. Bereavement is also distressing. Loss of family and friends causes pain, grief and loneliness, as well as loss of social role. However, death of a partner can provide the opportunity to learn new skills and develop new relationships.

> **remember**
>
> Human growth and development is affected in positive and negative ways by a range of factors and events.

Abuse

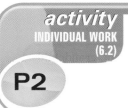 **link**

Links to Unit 2, pages 43–4.

---

activity
INDIVIDUAL WORK
(6.2)

P2

Interview an elderly friend or family member about the positive and negative influences on their lifelong growth and development.

---

activity
GROUP WORK
(6.3)

D1

Produce a display that explains how socialisation, socio-economic factors and life events can affect growth and development at each life stage.

Gender

As you know, society has expectations of the way men and women should look and behave, and life can be tough for people who don't feel comfortable with their birth gender. Unless they are confident about not meeting society's expectations, they may have a weak self-concept due to doubts about their self-image and value as an individual.

Family and relationships

Being in supportive, non-judgemental relationships with people helps build a strong self-concept. On the other hand, bullies who dominate, repress, ill-treat or neglect their family and friends cause them to doubt their self-image and lose their self-worth. Someone with a weak self-concept is at risk of becoming a bully in turn.

Abuse

Like bullying, abuse and self-abuse destroy people's self-esteem and make them question their self-image. Having low self-respect puts them at risk of further abuse, because they don't have the confidence or inner strength to defend themselves against an abuser or their own behaviour. Someone with a weak self-concept is at risk of becoming an abuser in turn.

Culture

As you know, racial discrimination means treating people who are culturally different less than fairly. Challenging people about their religious beliefs and practices, diet, style of dress, and so on, is disrespectful and can damage their self-image and self-worth.

Income

People on a low income may not be able to afford the things that bolster most people's self-concept, such as fashionable clothes, a car and up-to-date technological devices. If this troubles them, they may develop a weak self-concept. On the other hand, people on a higher income are more able to buy themselves a positive self-image. And being comfortably off usually goes hand in hand with high self-esteem.

remember	A variety of factors influence the development of self-concept.

Education

Education is a lifelong activity and every new thing we learn should be recognised as an achievement. Apart from making us more knowledgeable and interesting, improving our learning and understanding earns us respect from others and improves our self-confidence, self-image and self-esteem.

www.youth2youth.co.uk
www.more-selfesteem.com
www.troubledwith.com
www.self-confidence.co.uk
www.bbc.co.uk/health
www.netdoctor.co.uk

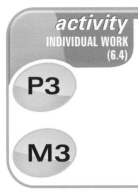

activity
INDIVIDUAL WORK
(6.4)

P3

M3

Describe five factors that have influenced the development of your self-concept.

The Changing Care Needs at Different Life Stages

This section looks at changing care needs and how health and social care workers can meet the needs of service users at different life stages.

Issues around life stages
Changing care needs at different life stages

You know now that we grow and develop physically, intellectually, emotionally and socially throughout our lives. Because of these changes, our care needs change. The table on page 144 shows how care needs can vary at different life stages.

link

Links to Unit 9, page 199.

activity
INDIVIDUAL WORK
(6.5)

P4

(a) Interview an elderly friend or family member about the care they have needed at different life stages.

(b) Write that person a letter that explains why their care needs have changed at different life stages.

Identifying, assessing and providing for needs

It's usually quite easy to identify when someone has physical care needs. Physical health care needs can be:

- acute, e.g. resulting from a viral infection, food poisoning or accidental injuries. People who work in the primary and secondary health care services, such as general practitioners (GPs), hospital doctors and nurses, identify, assess and provide for patients with acute physical needs.

- chronic health conditions that require ongoing, long-term care, e.g. asthma, diabetes and heart disease. People who work in the secondary health care services, such as specialist doctors and nurses, identify, assess and provide for patients with chronic physical needs.

Table 6.5 Changing care needs at different life stages

Life stage	Examples of care needs
Conception	Women who are trying to conceive have special physical health care needs, e.g. to eat a healthy diet that includes a folic acid supplement, to take regular exercise, to stop smoking, to cut back on alcohol and caffeine and to avoid stress. They also need emotional and social support.
Birth and infancy 0–3 years	During labour, mothers may need health care as well as emotional support; and their newborn babies may need special care, e.g. if they are premature or need help with their breathing. Babies and infants are totally dependent on their carers. • Physical care needs: a healthy diet, health care if necessary, toys and objects on which to practise their manipulative skills, room to develop their motor skills, and sensory stimulation. • Intellectual care needs: communication. • Emotional and social care needs: opportunities to bond and give and receive love and affection, security, praise and discipline.
Childhood 4–10 years	• Physical care needs: a healthy diet, room to play and health care if necessary. • Intellectual care needs: communication and opportunities to learn. • Emotional and social care needs: opportunities to develop relationships and give and receive love and affection, security, praise and discipline.
Adolescence 11–18 years	• Physical care needs: a healthy diet, regular exercise and health care if necessary. • Intellectual care needs: communication and opportunities to learn, become independent and think for themselves. • Emotional and social care needs: opportunities to develop new relationships and give and receive love and affection, security, praise, support and discipline.
Adulthood 19–65 years	Most adults are independent and have few care needs. However, some have special health care needs and some need support to live independently, work and to be responsible for themselves. And all adults need a healthy diet, regular exercise, opportunities to develop new relationships and give and receive love and affection, security and praise.
Old age 65+ years	All older people need security, a healthy diet, to stay as active as possible, opportunities to maintain relationships and give and receive love, affection and praise. Others have additional care needs. • Physical care needs: special health care and support with mobility, seeing and hearing as the body declines in function. • Intellectual care needs: support in keeping the mind active, communicating and maintaining memory. • Emotional and social care needs: support when they lose their independence and when friends and relatives pass away.
The final stages of life	People who are dying have very special health and care needs. They may need special medication and support in coming to terms with their future, particularly from close family and friends. Caring for people in the final stages of their life can be an exceptionally rewarding task.

Some people have care needs because they are physically disabled or have a sensory impairment. People with disabilities and impairments and their carers can apply for help to their local Social Services Departments, which will assess the degree of support they need and develop a care package describing how and by whom their needs will be met.

As you read in Unit 3, Social Services Departments work closely with other service providers to provide care and support, for example:

- the National Health Service, e.g. speech therapists and physiotherapists
- the voluntary sector, e.g. the Royal National Institute of the Blind (RNIB) and Scope, which works with people who have cerebral palsy
- the private sector, e.g. agencies that provide care and support to people in their own homes.

link

Links to Unit 3, pages 63–5 and Unit 8, pages 172–5.

Some people with intellectual care needs are described as having learning difficulties. Learning is difficult for people, for example, who have a chromosome disorder such as Down's syndrome, for people who have brain damage as a result of an accident and for people who suffered brain injury at birth.

A chromosome disorder can be identified during pregnancy through antenatal testing (screening). Learning difficulties caused by brain damage or injury are usually identified after the event by, for example, health care professionals, family, friends and school teachers. The needs of people with learning difficulties are met by Social Services Departments working in partnership with health care providers, education authorities, voluntary and private sector service providers, employers and carers.

As we get older, we can expect to develop intellectual care needs. We may find it difficult to make decisions on an everyday basis, live independently, manage our finances and take responsibility for ourselves and where we live. We can also expect that it will take longer to learn new things and be harder to remember recent events.

Elderly people don't always recognise that they have growing intellectual needs. Instead, friends and family, with the support of Social Services Departments, identify and assess the help they need. There is a range of services designed to help, for example care homes, day care and reminiscence therapy sessions provided by Social Services Departments, and private and voluntary groups such as Age Concern. There is also respite care, a service which gives carers an opportunity to have a break.

Figure 6.9
Meeting care needs

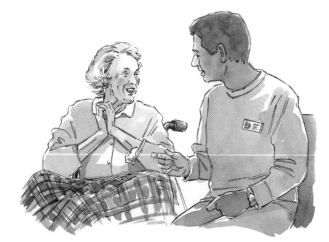

keyword

Self-refer
To choose for yourself to visit your GP, dentist, etc.

People with emotional care needs are often described as having mental health care needs. Someone experiencing stress, anxiety or depression can be referred by friends and relatives or can **self-refer** to their GP. GPs assess and treat patients or refer them on to mental health specialists for assessment. If a patient's care needs are assessed as being long term, mental health specialists will develop a care package that describes how and by whom the patient's needs will be met.

Mental health needs are met by professionals such as community mental health teams, aromatherapists and counsellors using, for example, medication, therapy and support. Care packages are reviewed on a regular basis, to ensure that they continue to deliver care that is appropriate and helpful.

As you read earlier, we begin to form relationships with people from the time we are born. However, people who are shy, embarrassed, don't know how to interact, or who are unable to communicate or get out and about find it hard to develop the social skills needed to build and maintain relationships. As a result, their behaviour may not be normal or acceptable and they may become lonely and socially isolated.

There is a range of services available for people who have social care needs, i.e. who are lonely, socially isolated or who need to develop social skills. For example, Social Services Departments, education authorities and voluntary and private organisations provide help and support through clubs for children and young people, family support groups, day centres and luncheon clubs.

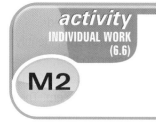

activity
INDIVIDUAL WORK (6.6)

M2

Think about the life events that you have experienced to date. Explain how they have affected your:

(a) development

(b) care needs.

Physical care

Health and social care workers meet service users' physical care needs by being alert to changes in their care needs, prompting a new care assessment if appropriate and by following care packages and workplace procedures so that care provided is safe and protective. This section describes how they can also meet service users' intellectual, emotional and social needs and improve their self-concept when giving physical care.

Respect

Health and care workers who are respectful, considerate and polite are likely to develop supportive and non-judgemental relationships with service users in which they feel valued and accepted for who they are.

Recognising diversity

Diversity is to do with the differences between people. We are all different because we have each been exposed to a different mix of socio-economic factors and life events. Health and social care workers have a responsibility to recognise service users' individual differences in the way they work with them, to ensure that they:

- treat them as individuals
- treat them with respect
- care for them in ways that meet their individual needs.

Dignity

Health and care workers who respect service users' dignity show that they value their beliefs about what is correct, their way of doing things and their way of presenting themselves. This strengthens their self-esteem and confidence in their self-image.

Active support

Health and care workers have a responsibility to actively help service users to stay independent. Promotion of independence encourages people to be responsible for themselves, to continue to achieve and feel fulfilled, and shows them that they are valued and respected for what they can and can't do. By actively supporting independence, health and care workers also ensure that they treat service users as individuals.

Health and care workers also have a responsibility to actively help service users make their own choices. Promotion of choice encourages people to stay in control of their lives and to continue to feel good about themselves. By actively supporting choice, health and care workers also ensure that they care for service users in ways that take account of their choices.

> **remember**
> As people grow and develop, their care needs change.

case study 6.3

Mrs Smith

Mrs Smith is a resident at a care home for elderly people. The staff are rude, prejudiced against elderly people, have never attempted to get to know Mrs Smith personally, are not bothered about helping her to look nice and don't give her an opportunity to do things for herself or to choose what to eat or wear.

activity
GROUP WORK

How do you think Mrs Smith feels?

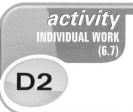

activity
INDIVIDUAL WORK
(6.7)

D2

Imagine that you are ill and need to stay in hospital for a couple of weeks. Explain how you would want to be cared for so that you retained your self-image and self-esteem.

The Department of Health www.dh.gov.uk
The Clinical Governance Support Team www.cgsupport.nhs.uk/Programmes

progress check

1. What are the main life stages?
2. Describe the main aspects of physical, intellectual, emotional and social development that take place at each life stage.
3. Explain the effects of three positive and three negative influences on human growth and development.
4. Explain the effects of three life events on human growth and development.
5. Describe five factors that can affect self-concept.
6. Explain why people have different care needs at different life stages.
7. Explain how meeting someone's care needs can help improve his or her self-concept.

Books

Clarke, L. (2002), *Edexcel Health and Social Care* GCSE (Nelson Thornes)

Fisher, A., Seamons, S., Wallace, I. and Webb, D. (2003), *GCSE Health and Social Care: Student Book* (Folens Publishers)

Gresford, P. (1997), *Case Studies in Health and Social Care* (Heinemann)

Lindon, J. (2002), *Early Years Care and Education* (Thomson Learning)

Mackean, D. G. (1988), *Human Life* (John Murray)

Mackean, D. G. and Jones, B. (1987), *Introduction to Human and Social Biology* (John Murray)

Meggitt, C. (1997), *A Special Needs Handbook for Health and Social Care* (Hodder Arnold)

Meggitt, C. and Bruce, T. (2002), *Child Care and Education* (Hodder Arnold)

Meggitt, C. and Sunderland, D. (2000), *Child Development: An Illustrated Guide* (Heinemann)

Meggitt, C. and Thomson, H. (1997), *Human Growth and Development for Health and Social Care* (Hodder Arnold)

Minett, P. (2001), *Child Care and Development* (John Murray)

Page, M. (ed) (2005), *The Human Body* (Dorling Kindersley)

Walsh, M. (2002), *Health and Social Care for GCSE: Teacher's Resource Pack* (Collins Educational)

Walsh, M. and De Souza, J. (2000), *Collins Health and Social Care for Intermediate GNVQ* (Collins Educational)

Windsor, G. and Moonie, N. (ed) (2000), *GNVQ Health and Social Care: Intermediate Compulsory Units with Edexcel Options* (Heinemann)

Wright, D. (2000), *Human Physiology and Health* (Heinemann)

Wright, D. (2001), *Human Physiology and Health for GCSE: Resource Pack* (Heinemann)

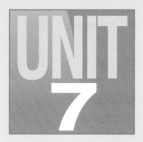

Creative and Therapeutic Activities in Health and Social Care

This unit covers:

- creative and therapeutic activities appropriate to users of different health and social care settings
- the potential benefits of creative and therapeutic activities for service users
- aspects of health and safety legislation, regulations and codes of practice relevant to the implementation of creative and therapeutic activities.

Creative and therapeutic activities have numerous benefits for service users in a wide range of health and social care settings. Health and social care workers need to understand the value of different activities, be able to choose activities that are appropriate to the individuals they are working with and know what measures to take in order to maintain health and safety. This unit gives learners an opportunity to develop an awareness of creative and therapeutic activities, understand their benefits and plan to carry out activities in a way that conforms with health and safety legislation.

grading criteria

To achieve a **Pass** grade the evidence must show that the learner is able to:	To achieve a **Merit** grade the evidence must show that the learner is able to:	To achieve a **Distinction** grade the evidence must show that the learner is able to:
P1 produce initial drafts and final plans for two different creative/therapeutic activities for different patients/service users in a health and social care setting Pg 169	**M1** explain how each creative/therapeutic activity could benefit the patient/service user Pg 164	**D1** recommend ways of improving each creative/therapeutic activity, taking into account individual needs Pg 164
P2 carry out and review the activities Pg 169	**M2** describe how health and safety issues were addressed for each creative/therapeutic activity Pg 168	**D2** explain why it was necessary to implement specific health and safety measures, linking these measures to the legislative requirements, regulations and codes of practice Pg 168
P3 identify potential benefits of the creative/therapeutic activity to the patient/service user Pg 164		

grading criteria

Creative and Therapeutic Activities Appropriate to Users of Different Health and Social Care Settings

keyword

Therapeutic
Healing.

Creative and **therapeutic** activities are carried out in a variety of different health and social care settings. This section describes some of those activities, where they take place and the service users that take part in them.

Health and social care settings

Figure 7.1

Where do creative and therapeutic activities take place?

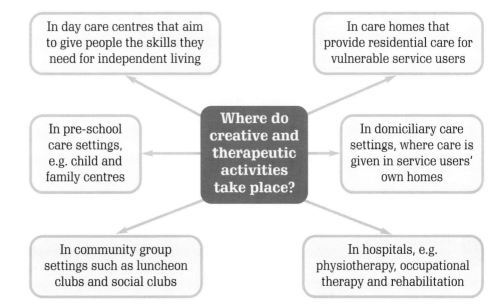

In day care centres that aim to give people the skills they need for independent living

In care homes that provide residential care for vulnerable service users

In pre-school care settings, e.g. child and family centres

Where do creative and therapeutic activities take place?

In domiciliary care settings, where care is given in service users' own homes

In community group settings such as luncheon clubs and social clubs

In hospitals, e.g. physiotherapy, occupational therapy and rehabilitation

Activities
Art and craft therapy

Art and craft therapy uses a wide variety of materials, for example paint, clay, dried flowers, shells, used greetings cards, and photographs. It allows service

keyword

Palliative care
Care which aims to kill pain.

users to express their thoughts and feelings visually, rather than in words. Art and craft therapists work in a variety of residential and community-based settings, with individuals and groups of children and elderly people experiencing stress, people with mental health problems and people with learning difficulties. They also work in hospices where **palliative care** is provided, and in prisons.

The British Association of Art Therapists www.baat.org

Drama therapy

Drama therapy uses techniques such as role play, mime and puppetry. It allows service users to tell their own story and express their feelings in ways that protect them from being criticised or judged. Drama therapists work in hospitals, schools, special schools and community centres with children, youths, adults and families under stress, people with mental health problems and people with learning difficulties.

The British Association of Dramatherapists www.badth.org.uk

Figure 7.2
Art and crafts

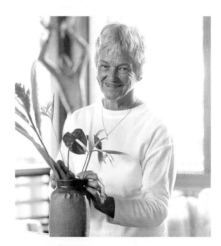

Role play

Role play allows service users who have difficulty using speech to express themselves through non-verbal communication techniques such as eye contact, facial expressions and gestures. It also helps service users who need to develop their non-verbal communication skills. Role play therapists work in a variety of settings with service users who, for example, stutter, have **dysphasia** and who lack confidence in their ability to communicate and develop relationships with others.

keyword

Dysphasia
The inability to use clear speech due to brain damage.

Music therapy

The music played in music therapy covers a wide range of styles and uses instruments that suit the needs of service users. It allows service users to express their feelings without using words and is not dependent on their having had any music training. Music therapists work with individuals and groups of people with learning disabilities, sensory impairments, and physical and emotional disorders. They work in a variety of settings such as hospitals, special schools, day centres, community centres and prisons.

The British Society for Music Therapy www.bsmt.org

Movement therapy

Movement therapy gives service users an opportunity to express their thoughts and feelings through movement such as dancing. Movement therapists work in day care settings, community centres and hospitals with a wide range of service users. They work with, for example, people who find it difficult to communicate using words, who are emotionally distressed, who have learning difficulties or who are ill or physically disabled.

The Association for Dance Movement Therapy UK www.admt.org.uk

Figure 7.3
Reminiscence therapy

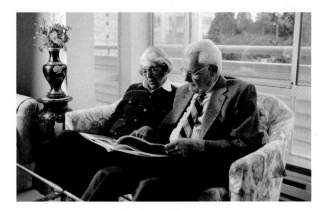

Reminiscence therapy

Reminiscence therapy encourages service users to talk about their experiences and the events that have happened in their lives. Reminiscence therapists usually work with groups of elderly people who have memory problems, using photographs, music and everyday items from the past to prompt their memory and help them evaluate their lives and possibly produce a book of their life story.

keyword

Reminiscence
Looking back, remembering.

Exercise therapy

Exercise therapy includes using gym equipment at health clubs and sports centres, going to exercise classes in community or day care settings, walking and cycling in the countryside and doing exercises at home. Service users who are referred to exercise therapy include people who are overweight, people who are depressed, elderly people, people with physical disabilities and people who are recovering from ill health.

Organising Medical Networked Information www.omni.ac.uk

Yoga therapy

Yoga therapy consists of exercises for posture, breathing and relaxation. It starts with very simple exercises so that service users can begin to practise and benefit right away, even if they have no experience. Yoga therapists work in community and day care centres, in care homes and domiciliary settings with individuals and groups of people who have a wide range of physical and emotional health conditions.

The British Council for Yoga Therapy www.yogatherapyforum.org.uk

Figure 7.4

Yoga therapy

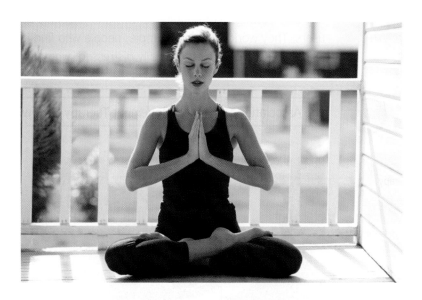

Writing therapy

Writing therapy is a form of self-help. It allows service users who have difficulty expressing themselves verbally to write down, in private, their thoughts and feelings about stressful events and traumatic experiences. It allows them, not professional workers, to choose the words that best describe how they feel and when and where to write their thoughts down. They can also choose whether to share their thoughts with anyone, rewrite them or destroy them.

Cooking

Cooking is a creative and skilled activity. It includes planning, food preparation, knowing about different methods of cooking, understanding cooking times and temperatures, using equipment and cleaning up. It also requires a knowledge of health, safety and hygiene. Cooking activities can be carried out by service users in any setting provided that equipment is appropriate and that supervision ensures safe, hygienic practice.

Therapeutic massage

Therapeutic massage involves manipulation of the body through gentle movements and pressure. It includes Indian head massage, which is carried out on the face, scalp, ears, neck, shoulders, arms and upper back; and on-site

keyword

Repetitive strain injuries
Injuries caused by repeating movements over and over again.

massage, which is carried out with the person sitting in a special, portable massage chair. Massage therapists work in a variety of settings with service users who have stress-related illnesses and physical problems such as back pain and **repetitive strain injuries**.

Figure 7.5
Cooking

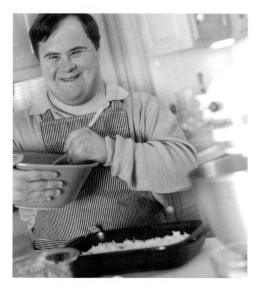

Games

Games are very important for service users at every life stage, whatever their ability or state of health. Games can be watched, for example football matches; and played, either alone or in a group. Games can be physical activities, played indoors, such as indoor bowls and darts, and outdoors, such as rounders and games at adventure playgrounds. And they can make people think, for example puzzles, quizzes, cards, board games and computer games. Games can be watched and played in any care setting that has the appropriate equipment and space.

Use of computers

Computers and the Internet can be installed in any care setting that has an electricity supply and a telephone connection. They can be used for a whole range of activities such as playing games, watching DVDs and TV, listening to music, keeping in touch with family and friends, sharing photographs, managing personal finances, shopping and studying courses. Adapted computers, such as touch screens, and specialist software, such as voice recognition software, make it easier for service users with physical disabilities, speech impediments, sensory impairments and learning difficulties to use and benefit from computer technology.

remember

There is a wide variety of creative and therapeutic activities appropriate to service users of different health and social care settings.

www.abilitynet.org.uk

activity
INDIVIDUAL WORK
(7.1)

Find out about five different creative and therapeutic activities that are carried out in social care settings and use your findings to complete the following table.

Table 7.1

Activity	Service user groups involved	Materials needed for each activity
1		
2		
3		
4		
5		

i

www.rethink.org
www.mentalhealth.org.uk
www.nhsdirectory.org
The NHS National Library for Health http://libraries.nelh.nhs.uk
www.helptheaged.org.uk
Speech and Language Therapy in Practice www.speechmag.com
www.speechteach.co.uk
www.learningdisabilities.org.uk
www.ability.org

The Potential Benefits of Creative and Therapeutic Activities for Service Users

This section looks at how appropriately chosen creative and therapeutic activities can benefit service users with a range of different needs.

The needs of service users
Physical needs

Many service users have physical care needs, for example they may have:

- stiff, swollen, painful joints, which affect their mobility and ability to use their hands

- stiff, sometimes rigid, muscles and tendons, which deform their limbs and make it difficult for them to be mobile and use their hands

- **involuntary** muscle movements, which make it difficult for them to control their movements

 keyword

Involuntary
Automatic, spontaneous, unintentional.

- poor circulation and respiratory problems, which cause tiredness and shortness of breath
- poor coordination and balance, which put them at risk of falling over
- weakness or paralysis in their left or right side, which make it difficult for them to carry out everyday tasks
- loss of a limb, which makes mobility and movement difficult.

Intellectual needs

Many service users have intellectual care needs, for example they may:

- have memory loss, caused by growing older or dementia, or because it is easier to deal with powerful emotions by pushing memories to the back of the mind; memory loss can be very frustrating
- have a learning difficulty or mental health problem, which makes it difficult for them to communicate effectively, behave appropriately, make decisions, solve problems, be responsible for themselves and live independently, etc.
- find it difficult to use language, for example if they have had a stroke and lost the ability to speak or if they have a speech impediment such as a stutter
- be bored and not interested in life around them.

Emotional needs

Many service users have emotional care needs, for example they may:

- have been separated from their loved ones, which can cause fear and anxiety
- have lost some or all of their independence, which can cause frustration and low self-confidence
- have negative feelings about their body image and the way others see them, which can cause low self-esteem
- have a medical condition or be taking medication that causes confusion, uncontrollable mood swings and distressing changes in behaviour
- be miserable and depressed.

Social needs

Many service users have social care needs, for example they may:

- be new to a care setting, which can make them feel lost, awkward and embarrassed
- be without friends, which can make them feel lonely and isolated
- feel neglected and abandoned by their family and friends, which can make it difficult to build new, trusting relationships.

case study 7.1 — New care settings

Barbara is approaching her 90th birthday and, because she is no longer able to look after herself at home, she has moved into a care home. The home is near her daughter but many miles away from where she has spent all her life.

Peter, who has been looked after by Social Services all his life, is having to leave his foster home and move into a flat with a view to developing independent living skills.

Jacob, who has an alcohol-related mental health condition, has been referred to a day care setting by his social worker.

activity
GROUP WORK

(a) What physical, intellectual, emotional and social needs do you think Barbara, Peter and Jacob have?

(b) How will their needs affect them?

The benefits of creative and therapeutic activities

Creative and therapeutic activities can help service users with physical, intellectual, emotional and social needs. They can also help them develop, maintain, improve and regain lost skills.

Developing new skills

Taking part in creative and therapeutic activities helps us to learn new skills, which gives us a sense of achievement and allows us to develop as individuals.

Service users in poor health or those who have a learning difficulty or disability are particularly likely to benefit from learning new skills. Learning new skills can promote their independence and improve their self-confidence, self-esteem and enjoyment of life. It can help them develop their ability to communicate and build friendships. It can also improve their ability to cope, reduce depression and help prevent mental conditions such as dementia.

Maintaining and improving current skills

Taking part in creative and therapeutic activities helps us to maintain and improve our skills, so that we continue to feel fulfilled and satisfied with life.

Age, disabilities and impairments affect service users' ability to do things. Many worry that their declining skills will have a negative effect on their independence and self-confidence in the future. Creative and therapeutic activities that enable them to practise and improve their skills help promote their independence and self-confidence, as well as maintain a sense of achievement, now and in the future.

Regaining lost skills

Figure 7.6
Lost skills

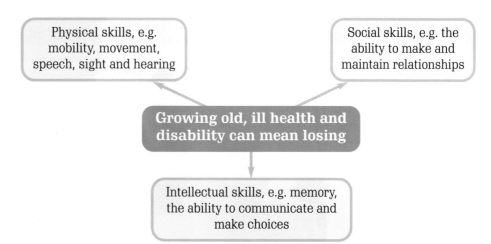

Losing the ability to do things can be distressing and demoralising. It can damage our self-concept and self-confidence, take away our independence and make us lonely and socially isolated. Creative and therapeutic activities give service users the opportunity to get back the skills they have lost, rebuild their self-esteem and self-image and promote their independence and social well-being.

Improving dexterity

Dexterity is to do with the physical ability to handle things. Disabling conditions such as arthritis make it difficult and sometimes painful to use our hands. It's also frustrating not to be able to do things with our hands; and people who lose dexterity lose a measure of independence.

Creative and therapeutic activities such as art and craft, writing, playing musical instruments and hand massage reduce tightness in the muscles and increase joint mobility. This helps service users to improve their dexterity, which in turn promotes their independence.

Improving fitness

Ill health, advancing age and disabilities affect our ability to stay mobile, which reduces our level of fitness. As we get less fit, our joints become rigid, our muscles become weak and stiff, we lose coordination and balance and we become breathless very easily.

Creative and therapeutic activities such as exercise, drama, movement, yoga and massage mobilise joints and relax and strengthen muscles, which helps improve coordination and balance. They also improve circulation and respiration, which helps reduce breathlessness. In other words, creative and therapeutic activities that promote fitness help service users to become more mobile, which in turn promotes their independence.

Figure 7.9

Creative and therapeutic activities that help raise self-esteem

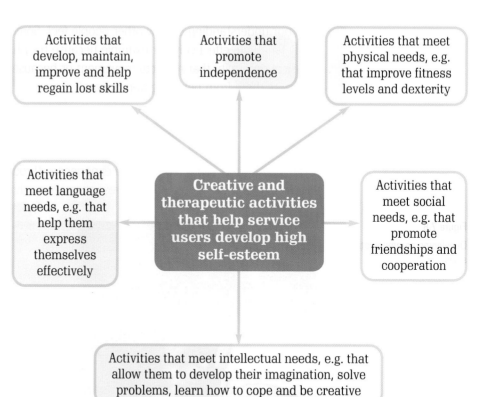

Choosing activities

When choosing creative and therapeutic activities, health and social care workers must have regard to a number of important issues.

Potential benefit and therapeutic value

There's no point choosing activities that won't benefit service users or have any therapeutic value for them. For example, art and craft sessions and writing therapy won't help people with extremely limited eyesight; and reminiscence therapy won't help people who are very deeply troubled by incidents in their past.

On the other hand, playing board games that use large-sized pieces will benefit people with dexterity problems, especially if they are competitive and like to win! And gentle exercise classes will help people who have difficulty moving, particularly if the session is fun and the participants supportive of each other.

Age

Our age affects the type of activities we know, enjoy and can do. When choosing creative and therapeutic activities, health and social care workers must bear service users' age in mind. For example, unless the elderly residents of a care home are keen to keep up with technology, there's no point investing in an Xbox to stimulate their minds! The youngsters in a children's home would probably be delighted if you did, but wouldn't be quite so pleased if you asked them to join you in a game of bezique or shove-ha'penny!

Cultural and social background

People from different social and cultural backgrounds have different customs, values and beliefs. For example, there are differences regarding the use of body language and touch, what to be called, how to dress and how to prepare and eat food. Health and social care workers need to think about social and cultural differences when choosing creative and therapeutic activities so that they don't cause offence or hurt people's feelings.

Gender

Our gender influences the type of creative and therapeutic activities that we are interested in and feel comfortable doing. For example, most men would rather watch a football match or play darts than spend time pressing flowers or cooking; and more women practise yoga and enjoy therapeutic massage than men. Health and social care workers need to think about gender differences when choosing creative and therapeutic activities in order to meet people's interests and prevent any embarrassment.

Service users' preferences

The most important consideration when choosing creative and therapeutic activities is service users' preferences. Unless they enjoy, feel comfortable with and can see the benefits of an activity, there is no point choosing it for them.

 Links to Unit 3, pages 66-8.

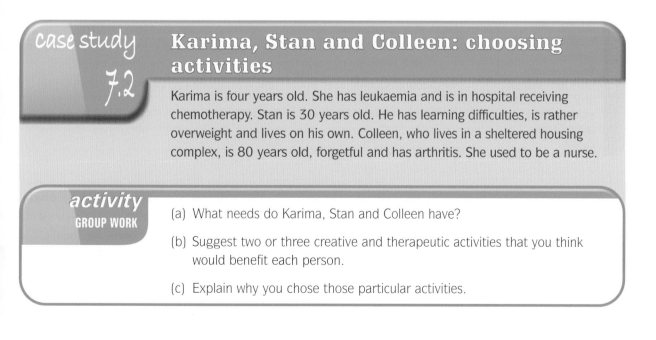

case study 7.2

Karima, Stan and Colleen: choosing activities

Karima is four years old. She has leukaemia and is in hospital receiving chemotherapy. Stan is 30 years old. He has learning difficulties, is rather overweight and lives on his own. Colleen, who lives in a sheltered housing complex, is 80 years old, forgetful and has arthritis. She used to be a nurse.

activity
GROUP WORK

(a) What needs do Karima, Stan and Colleen have?

(b) Suggest two or three creative and therapeutic activities that you think would benefit each person.

(c) Explain why you chose those particular activities.

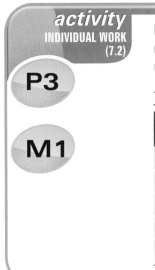

activity
INDIVIDUAL WORK
(7.2)

P3

M1

Look back at the five different creative and therapeutic activities that you researched for Activity 7.1. Complete the following table to demonstrate your understanding of their benefits to service users.

Table 7.2

Activity	Potential benefits to service users	Reasons why the activities can benefit service users
1		
2		
3		
4		
5		

Reviewing activities

Health and social care workers must review the creative and therapeutic activities they choose and carry out. They can do this by reflecting on:

- their choice of activity, i.e. was it appropriate for the service users involved, taking into account their individual preferences, age, gender and background?

- how they carried the activity out, i.e. did they give service users active support to do as much for themselves as possible, to maintain their independence? Did the activity meet individual service users' needs? And did they carry out activities in a way that conforms with health and safety legislation? You will read about health and safety in the next section.

remember

Creative and therapeutic activities can benefit service users with a range of different needs as long as they are appropriately chosen.

They should also seek feedback from other members of the care team, supervisors, NVQ assessors and, of course, service users, about how they might improve the activity for future use.

activity
GROUP WORK
(7.3)

D1

Geoff uses a wheelchair, is a vegetarian and has a pronounced stutter. He has just attended a cooking session at the day care centre he attends. He wasn't asked whether he would like to do the session: he was simply told that it had been organised and he was expected to join in. The dish that was being cooked was chicken curry. The kitchen is not adapted for wheelchair users. Geoff didn't enjoy the session: but the care worker who chose and led the activity didn't have time to wait for his feedback.

How could the activity have been improved for Geoff?

See the websites suggested in the previous section.

Aspects of Health and Safety Legislation, Regulations and Codes of Practice Relevant to the Implementation of Creative and Therapeutic Activities

Legislation, regulations and codes of practice

Service users have a right to be protected from danger and harm. This section describes the legislation, regulations and codes of practice that protect service users when they are taking part in creative and therapeutic activities.

The Health and Safety at Work Act (HASWA) 1974

The Health and Safety at Work Act 1974 is the most important workplace health and safety law. To uphold the rights of service users to be protected from danger and harm, health and social care workers have to obey the Health and Safety at Work Act 1974.

Food safety legislation

Because many service users are vulnerable, they are particularly at risk of food poisoning. To uphold their right to be protected from danger and harm, health and social care workers must follow workplace food-safety procedures when carrying out creative and therapeutic activities that involve food handling.

Figure 7.10

Health and social care workers' responsibilities under the HASWA

To take care of everyone they work with by:
- only doing activities for which they've been trained
- storing activity equipment safely and in the right place
- never fooling around with equipment

To report:
- health and safety hazards, e.g. activity equipment that is faulty and could cause an accident or injury
- accidents and injuries that happen whilst an activity is taking place

What are health and social care workers' health and safety responsibilities when carrying out creative and therapeutic activities?

To follow workplace health and safety procedures at all times

Health and social care workers have a responsibility to take part in health and safety training and to update their skills and knowledge when necessary. By doing so, they can be confident that they have the ability to uphold service users' rights to protection from danger and harm when carrying out creative and therapeutic activities.

activity

INDIVIDUAL WORK
(7.4)

P4

M2

Look back at the five different creative and therapeutic activities that you used to complete Activities 7.1 and 7.2. Now complete the following table to demonstrate your understanding of health and safety when carrying out creative and therapeutic activities.

Table 7.3

Activity	Relevant health and safety laws and regulations	How heath and safety issues should be dealt with
1		
2		
3		
4		
5		

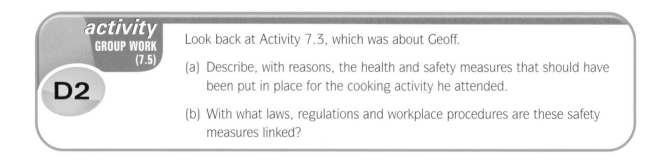

activity

GROUP WORK
(7.5)

D2

Look back at Activity 7.3, which was about Geoff.

(a) Describe, with reasons, the health and safety measures that should have been put in place for the cooking activity he attended.

(b) With what laws, regulations and workplace procedures are these safety measures linked?

activity
GROUP WORK
(7.6)

P1

P2

Choose one creative or therapeutic activity that you could use with a single service user and another that you could use with a group. Use different care settings and service users with different needs, for example a pre-school setting with a group of children and a care home setting with an elderly person.

For each activity produce a plan that identifies:

(a) the service user/s and why you have chosen to plan an activity for them (think about needs…)

(b) the activity and why you chose it (think about benefits and the appropriateness of the activity to service users…)

(c) what materials you need and how much of them

(d) when and where you would carry out the activity

(e) how you would maintain health and safety and why (think about legislation…).

Describe:

(f) how you would carry out the activity, step by step, giving as much detail as you can

(g) how you would review the activity.

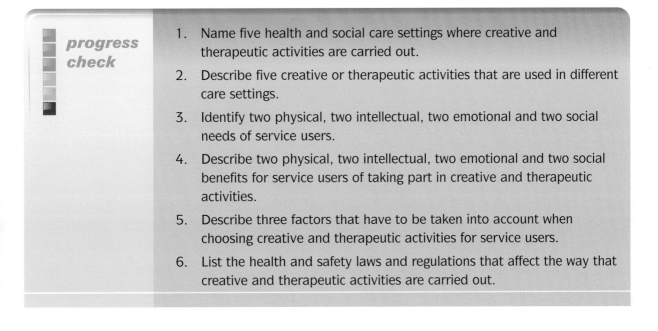

progress check

1. Name five health and social care settings where creative and therapeutic activities are carried out.

2. Describe five creative or therapeutic activities that are used in different care settings.

3. Identify two physical, two intellectual, two emotional and two social needs of service users.

4. Describe two physical, two intellectual, two emotional and two social benefits for service users of taking part in creative and therapeutic activities.

5. Describe three factors that have to be taken into account when choosing creative and therapeutic activities for service users.

6. List the health and safety laws and regulations that affect the way that creative and therapeutic activities are carried out.

Books

Barratt, C. (2000), *Intermediate Health and Social Care* (Oxford University Press)

Burnard, P. and Morrison, P. (1997), *Caring and Communicating* (Palgrave Macmillan)

Bruce, T. (2004), *Cultivating Creativity in Babies, Toddlers and Young Children* (Hodder Arnold)

Counsel and Care (1993), *Not only Bingo: Study of Good Practice in Providing Recreation and Leisure Activities for Older People in Residential Care and Nursing Homes* (Counsel and Care)

Court, C. (1993), *Festivals: Teachers' Timesavers Series* (Scholastic Ltd)

Hobart, C. and Frankel, J. (1999), *A Practical Guide to Activities for Young Children* (Nelson Thornes)

Meggitt, C. (1997), *A Special Needs Handbook for Health and Social Care* (Hodder Arnold)

Moonie, N. (2000), *Intermediate Health and Social Care* (Heinemann)

Moonie, N., Nolan, Y. and Lavers, S. (2003), *BTEC First Caring* (Heinemann)

Nazarko, L. (2000), *NVQs in Nursing and Residential Homes* (Blackwell Publishing)

Nolan, Y. (1998), *NVQ Level 2 in Care: Student Handbook* (Heinemann)

Skelt, A. (1993), *Caring for People with Disabilities* (Pearson)

Walsh, M. and de Souza, J. (2000), *Health and Social Care* (Collins)

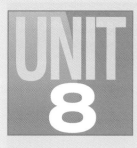

Health and Social Care Services

This unit covers:

- the organisation of health and social care service provision
- the potential benefits of working in partnership for health and social care service provision
- working in the health and social care sectors.

People who are thinking of working in health and social care need to know and understand how health and social care service providers are organised and how and why they work together. They also need to know about different job roles in the care sector and about career possibilities. This unit aims to give learners an opportunity to learn about health and social care services in England (links to services in Scotland, Wales and Northern Ireland are provided), the difficulties some people have in using those services and how working in partnership can improve the services provided. It also gives learners an opportunity to research the skills, requirements and developmental activities needed to maintain an effective and competent care workforce.

grading criteria

To achieve a **Pass** grade the evidence must show that the learner is able to:	To achieve a **Merit** grade the evidence must show that the learner is able to:	To achieve a **Distinction** grade the evidence must show that the learner is able to:
P1 describe the key elements of health and social care service provision in a named country Pg 179	**M1** use different examples to explain barriers to access of health and social care services Pg 181	**D1** explain how barriers to access to services may be overcome by effective partnership working Pg 185
P2 identify the factors that are potential barriers to access of health and social care services Pg 181	**M2** explain how the two examples of health and social care service providers working in partnership benefit patients/service users Pg 185	**D2** explain how workforce development activities help to maintain a competent health and social care workforce Pg 193

- planning for improved health services in their area
- increasing the number of services provided
- monitoring the performance and standards of local health care services.

Primary Care Trusts (PCTs)

PCTs control health care locally and are monitored by their SHA.

Figure 8.1

The functions of PCTs

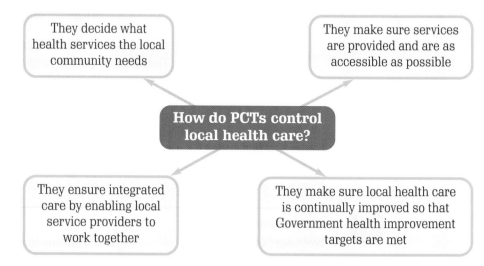

They decide what health services the local community needs

They make sure services are provided and are as accessible as possible

How do PCTs control local health care?

They ensure integrated care by enabling local service providers to work together

They make sure local health care is continually improved so that Government health improvement targets are met

Primary health care

Primary health care is the expression used to describe health services that are provided in the community. Primary health care service providers include family doctors (GPs), community and practice nurses, pharmacists, opticians, dentists, NHS walk-in centres and NHS Direct. They are the first, and sometimes only, contact that people have with the NHS.

Figure 8.2

Primary health care providers

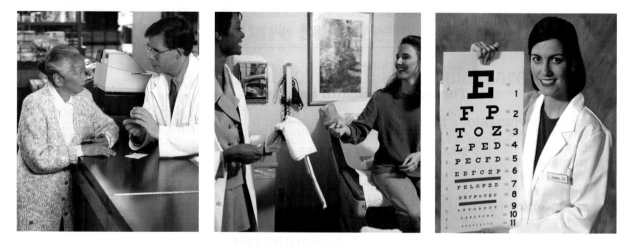

Secondary health care

Secondary health care is the expression used to describe health services that treat conditions not usually dealt with by primary health care providers. It includes:

■ acute (emergency) treatment

■ specialist medical treatment or surgery following a referral from a GP.

Secondary care is provided by NHS, children's, mental health, foundation and ambulance trusts.

Figure 8.3
Secondary health care providers

Children's trusts, which integrate health care, social care and education to improve the health and care of all children and young people

Mental health trusts, which provide treatment, therapy and specialist training for people with mental ill health in the community and in hospitals

Providers of secondary health care

NHS trusts run hospitals that provide free acute and specialist treatment. As well as working in hospitals, NHS trust employees work, e.g.:
■ in regional or national centres that provide very specialised care
■ at health centres, clinics and in people's homes
■ in universities, where they help to train health professionals

www.dh.gov.uk

The Scottish Executive www.scotland.gov.uk

The Department of Health for Northern Ireland www.dhsspsni.gov.uk

The NHS Wales www.wales.nhs.uk

www.nhs.uk

www.integratedcarenetwork.gov.uk

www.everychildmatters.gov.uk

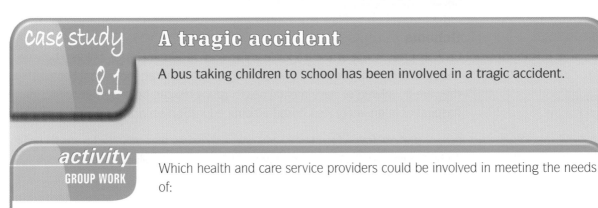

case study

8.1

A tragic accident

A bus taking children to school has been involved in a tragic accident.

activity

GROUP WORK

Which health and care service providers could be involved in meeting the needs of:

(a) everyone involved in the accident?

(b) parents, relatives and friends of the people involved in the accident?

Health and social care settings

Health and social care services are provided in a range of settings to meet the needs of a range of different service user groups and individuals.

Day nurseries

Day nurseries offer opportunities for children from about six weeks old to five years old to learn and develop through play. There are different types of day nursery, for example:

■ nurseries run by LAs and not-for-profit voluntary organisations
■ privately run businesses.

Some day nurseries follow the Foundation Stage of the National Curriculum. This enables staff to identify each child's achievements and plan to meet their learning and development needs.

Playgroups

Playgroups offer opportunities for children between the ages of about two and five to learn and develop through play. Some are run by LAs and voluntary organisations; some are run by parents; and others are privately run. Like nurseries, some playgroups follow the Foundation Stage of the National Curriculum.

Figure 8.4
Childcare settings

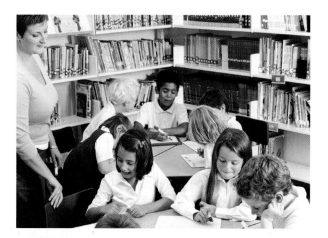

Schools

Schools provide opportunities for learning and development for children between the ages of four or five and eighteen. Pupils who can't attend school because they are ill, injured or have mental health problems can be taught at home, in hospital or in an integrated hospital/home education service.

School staff are trained to identify and deal with issues that can affect a child's health and well-being, such as shyness, learning difficulties and bullying. School nurses carry out health checks, such as hearing and sight tests, and give vaccinations. And pupils at schools follow the National Curriculum or a curriculum that suits their individual needs. By following a curriculum, teachers can measure pupils' learning and development and identify and provide for their individual needs.

Special schools

Special schools provide for pupils who have special educational needs. This means they have a learning difficulty that requires special provision to be made for them. Schools and LEAs work together to identify pupils' special educational needs and to provide them with the support they need. A pupil's Statement of Special Educational Needs describes their needs in detail and the special educational provision to be made for them.

Hospitals

As you read above, NHS hospitals provide acute and specialist treatment and surgery.

Figure 8.5

How hospitals meet needs

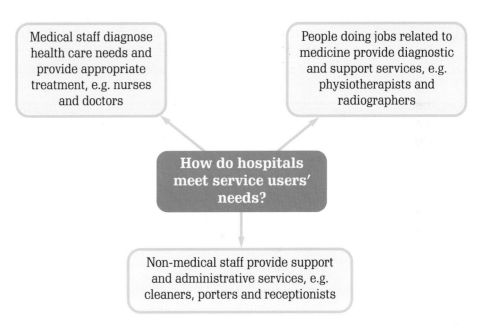

Medical staff diagnose health care needs and provide appropriate treatment, e.g. nurses and doctors

People doing jobs related to medicine provide diagnostic and support services, e.g. physiotherapists and radiographers

How do hospitals meet service users' needs?

Non-medical staff provide support and administrative services, e.g. cleaners, porters and receptionists

keyword

Decentralisation
Spread of control of services from central government to local government.

Foundation trusts are a new type of NHS hospital that are managed locally and meet the needs of the local population. They are an example of **decentralisation**.

Private hospitals provide a range of operations, treatments and investigations but don't usually provide acute care.

Care homes

Care homes provide round-the-clock care for people who:

- need care because of old age
- have dementia, mental illness or learning disabilities
- have physical disabilities or sensory impairment
- have past or present alcohol or drug dependence
- are terminally ill.

There are three main types of care home:

1. Homes without nursing, which provide help with personal care, e.g. bathing and dressing: they used to be called residential homes.

2. Homes with nursing: these used to be called nursing homes.

3. Homes that offer both residential and nursing care.

case study 8.2 — Choosing care homes

Mrs James is in good health but she is physically very frail and unable to look after herself properly. Her friend, Mrs Adams, has cancer. She is undergoing chemotherapy and is in a lot of pain. Another friend, Mrs Collins, has Alzheimer's. She neglects her appearance and diet, and forgets to take her medication. All three ladies currently live at home by themselves.

activity
GROUP WORK

What sort of care homes would meet their needs?

People can self-refer to a care home or they can request a needs assessment. This is carried out by a social worker from the LA Social Services Department. By talking to the person, the social worker identifies their needs, the problems they have, the help they have and the help they think they need. A care plan is the document that sums up the person's needs and describes how they will be met.

If someone is identified as needing 24-hour personal and/or nursing care, the social worker may refer them to a care home, where care is provided according to the instructions on the care plan.

Figure 8.6
Caring for adults

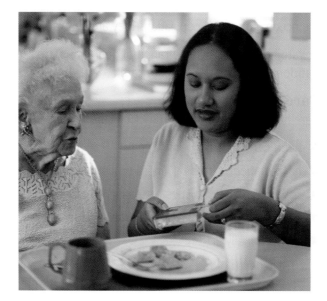

Links to Unit 6, pages 143–7.

Day centres

Service users are referred to day centres following a needs assessment. Day centres are usually located within the community and the services they provide include visits and activities that are aimed at helping service users maintain their independence. This in turn helps them to stay living in their own homes for as long as possible.

Domiciliary care

Domiciliary care is personal care provided to service users in their own home. People can make their own arrangements for personal home care or they can request a needs assessment. The needs assessment enables Social Services to work with other service providers to provide domiciliary care that meets the user's needs.

www.bbc.co.uk

www.childcarelink.gov.uk

The Inspectorate for Children and Learners in England www.ofsted.gov.uk

www.qca.org.uk

www.pre-school.org.uk

The Wales Pre-school Playgroups Association www.walesppa.org

The Scottish Pre-school Play Association www.sppa.org.uk

NIPPA – the Early Years Organisation www.nippa.org

The Training and Development Agency for Schools www.tda.gov.uk

www.teachernet.gov.uk

www.dfes.gov.uk/sickchildren

www.healthcarecommission.org.uk

www.csci.org.uk

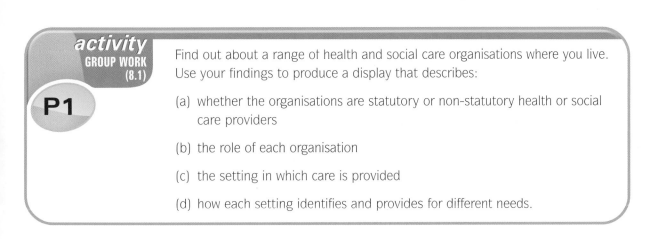

activity
GROUP WORK
(8.1)

P1

Find out about a range of health and social care organisations where you live. Use your findings to produce a display that describes:

(a) whether the organisations are statutory or non-statutory health or social care providers

(b) the role of each organisation

(c) the setting in which care is provided

(d) how each setting identifies and provides for different needs.

Access to health and social care services

In order to use health and care services, we have to know they exist and be able to:

- make contact with the people who work there
- visit the buildings in which the service is provided
- express our needs
- understand and carry out the instructions we are given.

Many people find it difficult to use health and social care services, as the following examples demonstrate.

Specific needs

Having specific needs can be a barrier to accessing services.

Table 8.1 Specific needs and barriers to accessing services

Examples of specific needs	How specific needs can be a barrier to accessing services
Mobility problems, e.g. people who use wheelchairs, crutches or walking frames	Difficult to use buildings, e.g. open doors, use steps and stairs
Disabilities, e.g. people with a speech impairment	Difficult to make themselves understood
Sensory impairments	Difficult to read directions and information, hear what is being said, fill in forms, etc.
Learning difficulties and emotional problems, e.g. embarrassment, anxiety, stress, depression, challenging behaviour	Difficult to communicate needs and understand what is being said
Different language	Difficult to read and understand information and express needs
Problems associated with growing old	Difficult to remember appointments or to take medication and to understand what is being said

Financial barriers

Telephoning and travelling to and from health and care services, car parking fees, prescriptions, home care, etc. can be very expensive for many people, even for those who receive financial help. As a result, people on a tight budget may think twice before accessing services.

Geographical barriers

Many people live in areas where service providers are not represented, where transport to and from a service provider is infrequent or non-existent or where service providers don't make home visits. As a result, they find it difficult to use services.

Social and cultural barriers

As you read in Unit 4, our social and cultural backgrounds and personal preferences mean that we have individual requirements and expectations about

> **remember**
>
> Health and social care services are provided by a range of organisations in a variety of settings but some are difficult to access.

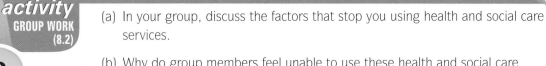
the way health and social care is provided. Unless our social, cultural and individual needs and preferences are respected by service providers, many of us would feel uncomfortable with the care we are given and unable to use services.

activity
**GROUP WORK
(8.2)**

P2

M1

(a) In your group, discuss the factors that stop you using health and social care services.

(b) Why do group members feel unable to use these health and social care services? Give examples.

 link

Links to Unit 4, pages 78–90.

The Potential Benefits of Working in Partnership for Health and Social Care Service Provision

You read earlier that the NHS, local authority Social Services Departments, and voluntary and private organisations work together with the aim of improving the services they provide. This is called partnership working.

Examples of working in partnership
Multi-agency working

Multi-agency working is about bringing together practitioners with a range of skills to work together as a team.

www.everychildmatters.gov.uk
www.ageconcern.org.uk
www.elderabuse.org.uk
The British Geriatrics Society www.bgs.org.uk
www.standards.dfes.gov.uk
www.dyslexia-inst.org.uk
www.scope.org.uk
www.downs-syndrome.org.uk
www.connexions.gov.uk

Table 8.2 Multi-agency working

Examples of services where multi-agency working takes place	Practitioners involved
Child protection	Social workers, teachers, health care workers, educational psychologists, education welfare officers, family support workers, police officers, etc.
Youth offending (drugs and alcohol)	Substance misuse workers, education welfare officers, probation officers, community psychiatric nurses, police officers, social workers, Citizens Advice Bureaux, Connexions, domestic abuse workers, etc.
Elder abuse	Geriatricians, GPs, nurses, social workers, care workers, voluntary organisations, such as Age Concern, Action on Elder Abuse and the British Geriatrics Society, police officers, etc.
Community care	Social workers, care workers, doctors, nurses, health visitors, occupational therapists, physiotherapists, voluntary organisations, etc.
Learning difficulties and behavioural problems	Learning mentors, teachers, educational psychologists, counsellors, social workers, specialist health care professionals, voluntary organisations, such as the Dyslexia Institute, SCOPE and the Down's Syndrome Association, Connexions, family support workers, etc.

Service users/carers involved in planning/decision making

As you know, when someone applies to receive care from LA Social Services Departments, a social worker has to assess that person's needs and produce a care plan. Care plans should be reviewed on a regular basis and amended to take account of service users' changing needs.

Service users have a right to be cared for in ways that take account of their choices. They also have a right to say how they want to be cared for. For this reason, they should be involved in assessing their needs, deciding how their needs will be met and reviewing their care plans.

Carers know a great deal about the interests, abilities and personal preferences of the people they care for. For this reason, they too should be involved in care needs assessment, care planning and care plan review.

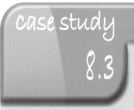

case study 8.3   Mr Hazell's care needs

A social worker has come to assess Mr Hazell's care needs. His wife, who is his main carer, is not asked to be present and the social worker tells Mr Hazell what she thinks his needs are and how she thinks they may be best met.

activity
GROUP WORK

Why is this an example of bad practice?

PCTs liaising with other organisations

Figure 8.7
PCTs working in partnership

NHS trusts, to help them raise their standards high enough to become Foundation trusts. Locally managed Foundation trusts are able to meet the needs of the local population better than Government-controlled NHS trusts

Social services, to help people who need care that isn't provided by health care services, e.g. Sure Start, which aims to improve the health of children through childcare and family support

PCTs liaise with

Local university departments, with whom many PCTs carry out research projects. The aim of their research is to improve primary and community care by finding new drugs and therapies

Representatives from **charitable** (voluntary) **organisations**, to improve the experiences of carers and of service users on whose behalf the charities work

The purpose of working in partnership

You now know that partnership working aims to develop health and social care services that meet people's needs, improve the way care is provided and improve the experiences of people using the services. This section describes how partnership working benefits both service users and health and care workers.

The holistic approach

By working together, different health and social care organisations are able to provide **holistic care**.

Because holistic care is about meeting individual needs, it respects a person's right to be treated as an individual. It improves their experience of being cared for, increases their emotional and social well-being and preserves their dignity.

keyword

Holistic care
Care that meets all of a person's physical, intellectual, emotional and social needs.

they protect children at risk, arrange foster care and adoption; they support young adults to live independently; and they help parents who can't cope. They also work with adults, assessing their care needs and developing care plans. Some social workers work with offenders.

Residential social workers work with residents in care homes, children's homes, hostels and youth centres. They assess needs, give social and emotional support, organise leisure activities, help with daily living activities and make sure that service users are safe and treated with dignity.

Youth workers

Many youth workers work in youth clubs or activity centres, for example sports clubs and drama centres. They talk to young people about a range of issues such as health, education, offending, volunteering and homelessness. Some are known as 'detached workers'. They meet young people on the street, in cafés and shopping centres, to offer advice and help.

Family support workers

Family support workers help and support families who are experiencing problems such as disabilities, behavioural problems, drug and alcohol abuse or where a parent is in hospital or in prison. Their aim is to help keep children with their families rather than being taken into care. In crisis situations, for example when a child is abandoned in the home or a single parent goes into hospital, family support workers can move into the child's home until alternative care is found.

Nurses

Nurses work in one of four areas: with children, adults, learning disabilities or mental ill health. They work in hospitals and in the community, for example in schools, walk-in centres and clinics. They give practical nursing care, including making routine measurements and observations, assisting doctors with physical examinations, giving drugs and injections, cleaning and dressing wounds and administering blood transfusions and drips.

Learning disability nurses support service users by teaching them skills and giving them the confidence they need to be as independent as possible. Mental health nurses give medication, support and counselling, and physical care if service users are too old or ill to look after themselves.

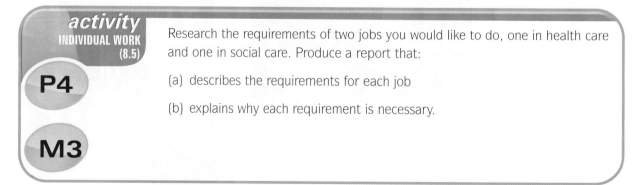

activity
**INDIVIDUAL WORK
(8.5)**

P4

M3

Research the requirements of two jobs you would like to do, one in health care and one in social care. Produce a report that:

(a) describes the requirements for each job

(b) explains why each requirement is necessary.

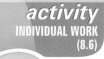

activity
INDIVIDUAL WORK
(8.6)

P5

Produce an information leaflet that describes the skills needed for the two jobs you found out about for Activity 8.5.

Workforce development

Thousands of people take part in learning every year, some for personal interest and others to gain qualifications or skills that will improve their job prospects and self-confidence. The health and social care sectors promote learning and development because an educated, skilled workforce goes hand in hand with a high level of service.

Health and care workers should identify their own learning and skills needs, through reflecting on and reviewing their performance. They should also ask their colleagues and supervisors to monitor their performance and give them feedback. Feedback can be on the job and in private, for example during appraisals. Feedback sessions are opportunities to agree and record workers' learning and skills needs and plan for their development.

> **keyword**
>
> **Qualification frameworks**
> A set of qualifications at different levels.

The Sector Skills Councils Skills for Health and Skills for Care and Development work with the health and social care sectors respectively. Their purpose is to develop the learning and skills of the care workforce with a view to improving care services. To do this they produce **qualification frameworks** that meet workers' continuing professional development (CPD) needs, allowing them to progress their careers. You read about CPD in Unit 3.

National occupational standards (NOS), which are developed by the health and social care Sector Skills Councils, describe what needs to be done in the workplace. Workers can demonstrate their continuing professional competence by achieving NVQs (SVQs in Scotland).

Skills for Care requires new social care workers to take part in an induction process. You read about this in Unit 3. Induction teaches workers how to provide high-quality care and prepares them for S/NVQs and other health and social care qualifications. It also helps them to become registered.

link

Links to Unit 3, page72.

Agenda for Change is a scheme for NHS workers that encourages them to take part in professional development. All job roles within the NHS have been assessed for skills, knowledge and responsibilities and are matched to a point on a pay band. As staff develop their skills and knowledge, they are rewarded by being moved up the pay band. The NHS Knowledge and Skills Framework identifies the knowledge and skills they need to use in their jobs, guides them in their learning and development and is used to determine their position on the pay band.

The skills escalator lets NHS workers develop their skills and knowledge at the next level up, in readiness for promotion. As a result, their careers are more satisfying and challenging, they are prepared for new jobs and the NHS has a pool of workers to replace staff who leave and to staff new services.

Figure 8.12

The skills escalator

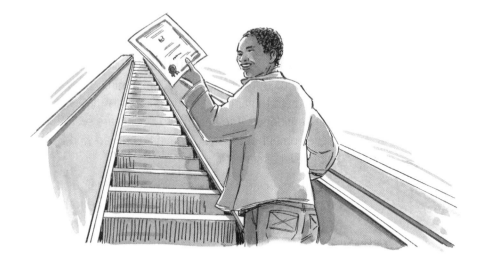

Succession planning is where employers identify workers' abilities and provide staff development programmes that allow them to progress their careers. Like the skills escalator, succession planning encourages workers to develop their skills and knowledge but it also meets the needs of the organisation by retaining experienced people.

Guidance

Figure 8.13

Developing in your job

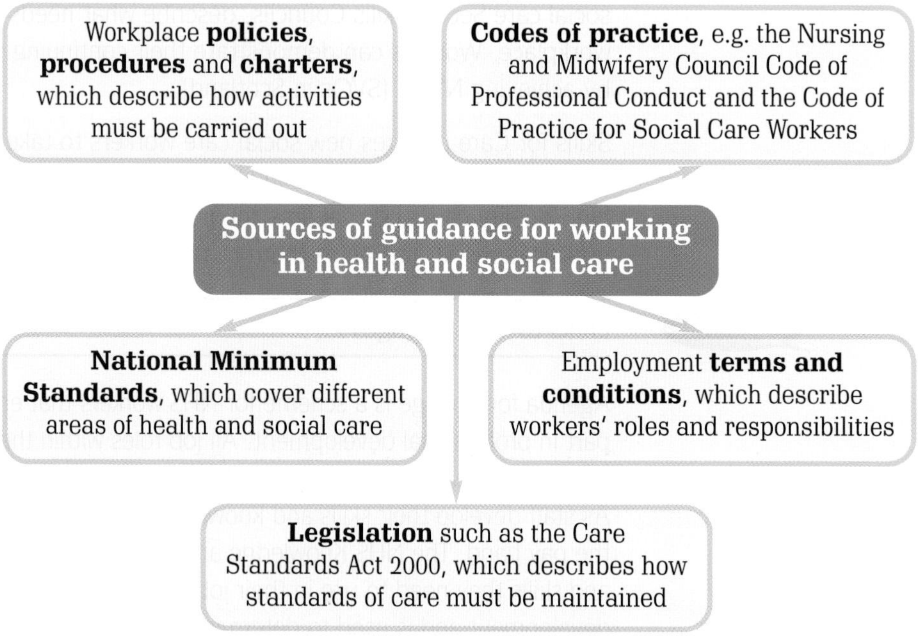

Workplace **policies**, **procedures** and **charters**, which describe how activities must be carried out

Codes of practice, e.g. the Nursing and Midwifery Council Code of Professional Conduct and the Code of Practice for Social Care Workers

Sources of guidance for working in health and social care

National Minimum Standards, which cover different areas of health and social care

Employment **terms and conditions**, which describe workers' roles and responsibilities

Legislation such as the Care Standards Act 2000, which describes how standards of care must be maintained

case study 8.4 — Aisha's future

Aisha has been a part-time assistant in the kitchen at your workplace for a number of years. She is thinking about becoming a full-time cook, nursing assistant or care worker. She doesn't know very much about these job roles.

activity — GROUP WORK

Where could Aisha find information and guidance that would help her make a decision about her future?

www.dfes.gov.uk/childrenswfqualifications
The National Youth Agency www.nya.org.uk
www.skillsforhealth.org.uk
www.skillsforcare.org.uk
The Health Protection Agency www.hpa.org.uk
www.socialcaring.co.uk
www.unison.org.uk
The Nursing and Midwifery Council www.nmc-uk.org
www.gscc.org.uk
www.learning.wales.gov.uk
The Care Standards Inspectorate for Wales www.csiw.wales.gov.uk
The Northern Ireland Assembly www.niassembly.gov.uk
www.scotland.gov.uk
www.niscc.info

> **remember**
> There is a huge variety of skilled work in the health and social care sector and numerous opportunities for professional and personal development.

activity — INDIVIDUAL WORK (8.7)

P6

Look back at the two job roles you researched for Activity 8.5.

(a) Where might workers in these jobs find guidance about how to progress their careers?

(b) What could they do to develop themselves as workers?

M4

(c) Give three reasons why it is important that health and social care workers develop themselves.

activity — GROUP WORK (8.8)

D2

Produce a display entitled 'The role of workforce development in maintaining a competent health and social care workforce'.

progress check

1. Describe three health care services and three social care services provided by the health and social care systems in the country where you live.

2. Describe the settings in which these health and social care services are provided.

3. List five factors that can prevent people accessing health and social care services.

4. Explain how these factors prevent people accessing services.

5. Describe two ways in which health and social care providers work together.

6. Explain how these partnerships benefit service users.

7. Explain the skills and requirements needed for a receptionist, a cleaner in a health or care setting, a health care assistant and a care worker.

8. How could each of these four workers develop themselves in readiness for promotion?

9. Why is it important that health and care workers continue to develop themselves?

Books

Clarke, L. (2002), *Edexcel Health and Social Care GCSE* (Nelson Thornes)

Fisher, A., Seamons, S., Wallace, I. and Webb, D. (2003), *GCSE Health and Social Care: Student Book* (Folens Publishers)

Moonie, N. (2000), *Intermediate Health and Social Care* (Heinemann)

Moonie, N., Nolan, Y. and Lavers, S. (2003), *BTEC First Caring* (Heinemann)

Richards, A. (1999), *The Complete A–Z Health and Social Care Handbook* (Hodder Arnold)

Walsh, M. (2002), *Health and Social Care for GCSE: Teacher's Resource Pack* (Collins Educational)

Walsh, M. and De Souza, J. (2000), *Collins Health and Social Care for Intermediate GNVQ* (Collins Educational)

Windsor, G. and Moonie, N. (ed) (2000), *GNVQ Health and Social Care: Intermediate Compulsory Units with Edexcel Options* (Heinemann)

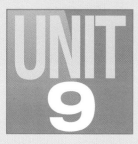

UNIT 9

The Impact of Diet on Health

This unit covers:

- the dietary needs of individuals at different life stages
- the effects of unbalanced diets on the health of individuals
- specific dietary needs of service users
- the principles of food safety and hygiene.

To help maintain or improve their own health as well as that of the people they work with, health and social care workers need to understand the importance of a balanced diet and how diet affects health. They need to know and understand the dietary requirements of individuals at different life stages and of service users with specific needs. They also need to know and use good practice in relation to food safety and hygiene.

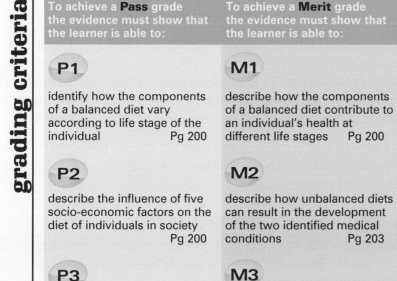

grading criteria

To achieve a **Pass** grade the evidence must show that the learner is able to:	To achieve a **Merit** grade the evidence must show that the learner is able to:	To achieve a **Distinction** grade the evidence must show that the learner is able to:
P1 identify how the components of a balanced diet vary according to life stage of the individual Pg 200	**M1** describe how the components of a balanced diet contribute to an individual's health at different life stages Pg 200	**D1** explain why the components of a balanced diet vary according to life stage of the individual Pg 200
P2 describe the influence of five socio-economic factors on the diet of individuals in society Pg 200	**M2** describe how unbalanced diets can result in the development of the two identified medical conditions Pg 203	**D2** explain how the two-day diet plan meets the dietary needs of the patients/service users Pg 208
P3 identify two medical conditions related to unbalanced diets Pg 203	**M3** describe why the identified specific dietary needs require dietary adjustment for the two patients/service users Pg 208	

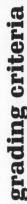

grading criteria

To achieve a **Pass** grade the evidence must show that the learner is able to:	To achieve a **Merit** grade the evidence must show that the learner is able to:	To achieve a **Distinction** grade the evidence must show that the learner is able to:
P4 produce a two-day diet plan for two patients/service users with specific dietary needs Pg 208	**M4** describe the effects of unsafe practices when preparing, cooking and serving food Pg 213	
P5 identify the safe practices necessary in preparing, cooking and serving food Pg 213		

The Dietary Needs of Individuals at Different Life Stages

Concept of a balanced diet

'Diet' is the word used to describe the type and amount of food we eat on a daily basis. The term 'balanced diet' describes the type and amount of food we need to eat to stay healthy and avoid **malnutrition**.

keyword

Malnutrition
A condition caused by not eating a balanced diet, eating too much or not eating enough.

Food supplies the body with energy to function and be active. Eating too much (overnutrition) or not eating a balanced diet upsets the energy balance. Unless excess energy is used up, for example in physical activity, overeating leads to ill health caused by being overweight. On the other hand, too low an intake of food can lead to undernutrition, nutritional deficiency diseases and starvation.

Dietary Reference Values (DRVs) give guidance about the energy and food requirements of different people at different life stages. You will read about individual dietary needs and the effects of unbalanced diets shortly.

The balance of good health

Although people's dietary needs vary, the types of food we should eat on a daily basis fall into five groups. To achieve a healthy balance, we should eat them in the following relative proportions:

■ plenty of bread, other cereals and potatoes

■ plenty of fruit and vegetables

■ moderate amounts of meat, fish and alternatives

Figure 9.1

Not a balanced diet!

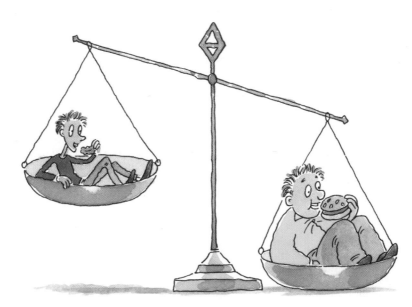

■ moderate amounts of milk and dairy foods

■ small amounts of fatty and sugary foods.

In addition, we should enjoy our food, eat a variety of different foods, eat the right amount to be a healthy weight and take in at least one litre of water every day.

 Links to Unit 2, pages 45–6.

Components of a balanced diet

The table on the following page describes the nutrients (components of food) that are needed for a balanced diet. These are **macronutrients** and **micronutrients**.

> **keyword**
>
> **Macronutrients**
> Nutrients that the body needs in large amounts, e.g. carbohydrates.

The body is about two-thirds water. Water is necessary for almost all body processes to take place; it is lost from the body in urine, sweat, faeces and exhaled air and must be replaced through our diet. Without water, we would become dehydrated and live for only a few days.

You read above that we should take in at least one litre of water every day. Both food and beverages (drinks) provide us with water. The exact amount we need depends on, for example:

> **keyword**
>
> **Micronutrients**
> Nutrients that the body needs in trace (small) amounts, e.g. some vitamins and minerals.

■ the temperature and our level of activity: water lost through sweating needs to be topped up

■ our diet, e.g. salty food increases the body's need for water

■ our age. Infants and young children have a greater need for water than adults.

Table 9.1 The components of a balanced diet

Nutrients in a balanced diet	Food sources	Role in the diet
Carbohydrates There are three types of carbohydrate in food: sugar, starch and fibre. Sugars are simple molecules and easily digested. Starch and fibre are complex molecules. Starchy foods need to be cooked before digestion can break them down to sugars, and fibre cannot be digested.	Sources of sugars include milk, fruit and fruit juice, table sugar; and food made using sugar, e.g. sweets, cakes, biscuits, chocolate and ice cream. Sources of starch include potatoes, yams, cereals, e.g. wheat, corn and oats; and food made using cereals, e.g. breakfast cereals, bread and cakes. Sources of fibre include fruit and vegetables and food made using bran, e.g. wholemeal bread and breakfast cereals.	Sugars and starch provide energy. Fibre adds bulk to the faeces, helping prevent constipation.
Proteins During digestion, protein breaks down into amino acids. The body can make some of the amino acids it needs; those it can't make are called essential amino acids and have to be present in the food we eat.	Animal sources include meat, fish, milk, cheese and eggs. Plant sources include peas, beans, nuts, cereals and seeds. Protein alternatives include tofu, miso and Quorn. It is important that vegetarians and vegans eat a varied diet, to make sure they take in enough essential amino acids.	Proteins are needed for growth and repair of the body and for energy.
Fats and **oils** During digestion, fats and oils break down to form glycerol and fatty acids. Fatty acids can be saturated, unsaturated and polyunsaturated. Saturated fatty acids (in fats) are linked with high cholesterol levels and CHD; unsaturated fatty acids (in oils) are linked with good health.	Fat is found in animal products such as lard, dripping, butter, meat and cheese; and in foods made using fat, e.g. cakes, biscuits and chocolate. Oil is found in plant products such as vegetable oils, nut oils, e.g. peanuts, fish oils, e.g. mackerel and tuna; and in foods made using oils, e.g. margarine.	Fats and oils provide energy and, when converted into body fat, keep us warm.
Vitamins: **A**, **B**, **C**, **D**, **E** and **K**	Vitamins are found in a variety of foods, including fresh fruit and vegetables, meat, fish, milk, eggs, margarine and breakfast cereals.	Vitamins are necessary for general good health, e.g. A helps us see in the dark; C maintains healthy skin and gums and helps wounds to heal; D makes bones strong; and K is necessary for the blood to clot.
Minerals: **calcium**, **sodium**, **iron** and **potassium**	Minerals are found in a variety of foods, including vegetables, meat, milk, table salt and foods containing salt.	Calcium is needed for strong bones and teeth; sodium for maintaining the body water level; iron to enable blood to carry oxygen; and potassium for muscles and nerves to function.

Diet variation during life stage development

Babies and infants (0–3 years)

Breastfeeding or formula milk, along with extra drinks of water in hot weather, meet a baby's nutritional needs for the first four to six months. At about six months, a baby can be weaned onto, for example, infant cereals and puréed fruit and vegetables. By the age of one and a half, whilst milk still plays an important role in their diet, infants are able to eat the same food as the rest of the family.

Children (4–10 years) and adolescents (11–18 years)

Children and adolescents grow quickly and are very active. They have big appetites and high nutritional needs. In particular, they need plenty of high energy and growth foods such as bread, potatoes, milk, cheese, meat, fish, fruit and vegetables.

They are also at a stage when unhealthy snack foods are tempting and when body image is important. Developing sensible eating habits is important for weight management and prevention of illness in adulthood due to obesity and underweight.

Adults (19–65 years)

Adults are usually less active than children and adolescents and so have lower nutritional needs. In general, they should eat appropriate amounts of a variety of foods from the five groups you read about earlier. An 'appropriate amount' depends on, for example:

- activity levels. Someone who leads an active lifestyle or has a physically demanding occupation will need more energy and protein foods than someone who sits in front of a TV or computer screen for long periods.

- weight. Someone who is managing their weight by going on a weight-reducing diet will eat smaller amounts of fats and sugars.

Women who are pregnant and breastfeeding have additional nutritional needs. Their diet needs to contain plenty of energy, protein, iron, calcium, folic acid, vitamins C and D and water to provide for the growth and development of the baby, changes in the mother's body and energy to carry the extra weight.

Old age (65+ years)

As people age, they become less active and have smaller appetites. Their need for energy food declines but they still require protein, fats, fibre, vitamins and minerals in amounts to satisfy their hunger.

link

Links to Unit 6, page 144.

Figure 9.2

A meal the whole family can enjoy

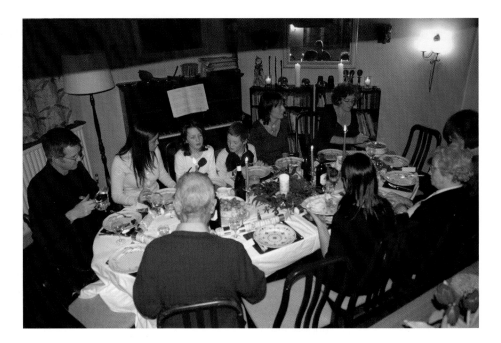

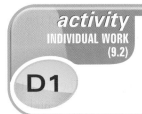

activity
GROUP WORK
(9.1)

P1

M1

(a) Produce a series of images, e.g. plates of food, food pyramids, that show what people should be eating at different stages of their life.

(b) Use your images to describe how the components of a balanced diet help people at different life stages to stay healthy.

activity
INDIVIDUAL WORK
(9.2)

D1

Produce a health education leaflet that explains why people need to vary their diet as they progress through life.

Factors influencing the diet of individuals

Figure 9.3

Socio-economic factors that affect people's diet

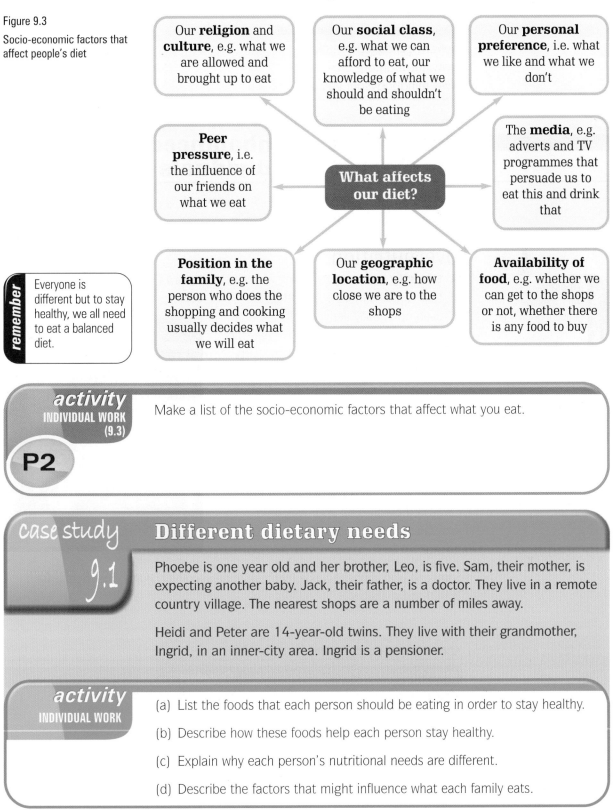

Our **religion** and **culture**, e.g. what we are allowed and brought up to eat

Our **social class**, e.g. what we can afford to eat, our knowledge of what we should and shouldn't be eating

Our **personal preference**, i.e. what we like and what we don't

Peer pressure, i.e. the influence of our friends on what we eat

What affects our diet?

The **media**, e.g. adverts and TV programmes that persuade us to eat this and drink that

Position in the family, e.g. the person who does the shopping and cooking usually decides what we will eat

Our **geographic location**, e.g. how close we are to the shops

Availability of food, e.g. whether we can get to the shops or not, whether there is any food to buy

remember

Everyone is different but to stay healthy, we all need to eat a balanced diet.

---

activity

INDIVIDUAL WORK (9.3)

P2

Make a list of the socio-economic factors that affect what you eat.

---

case study 9.1

Different dietary needs

Phoebe is one year old and her brother, Leo, is five. Sam, their mother, is expecting another baby. Jack, their father, is a doctor. They live in a remote country village. The nearest shops are a number of miles away.

Heidi and Peter are 14-year-old twins. They live with their grandmother, Ingrid, in an inner-city area. Ingrid is a pensioner.

---

activity

INDIVIDUAL WORK

(a) List the foods that each person should be eating in order to stay healthy.

(b) Describe how these foods help each person stay healthy.

(c) Explain why each person's nutritional needs are different.

(d) Describe the factors that might influence what each family eats.

www.food.gov.uk
www.nutrition.org.uk
www.eatwell.gov.uk/healthydiet
www.helptheaged.org.uk
www.nutrition.org.uk
www.mindbodysoul.gov.uk

The Effects of Unbalanced Diets on the Health of Individuals

You read earlier that malnutrition results from not eating a balanced diet. This section describes some common medical conditions associated with malnutrition.

Overnutrition

> **keyword**
>
> **Obesity**
> An excessive amount of body fat.

- **Obesity** is caused by eating a diet that contains more energy than is used up in daily activities. If we don't use the energy in the food we eat, the food is converted into body fat. Fatty and sugary foods contain the most energy and are the most fattening, but protein and other types of carbohydrate can also be turned into body fat.

Body Mass Index (BMI) is used to assess whether someone is overweight. It is calculated by dividing your weight in kilograms by the square of your height in metres.

Someone who is obese has a high risk of developing coronary heary disease (CHD) and diabetes.

Figure 9.4
Obesity

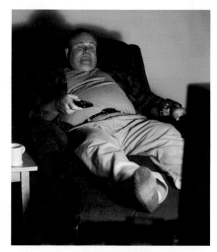

Table 9.2 BMI as a guide to health

BMI	Comment
Less than 18.5	Underweight
18.5–24.9	Ideal
25–29.9	Overweight
30–40	Obese
More than 40	Very obese

Coronary arteries
Blood vessels that
supply the heart
muscle with blood.

keyword

- **Coronary heart disease (CHD)**. You read in Unit 5 that a fatty diet is one of the causes of CHD. This is because saturated fatty acids in fat can increase the amount of cholesterol in the blood, which is deposited as plaques on artery walls. As plaques build up in the **coronary arteries**, the amount of blood reaching the heart is reduced, causing coronary heart disease. Heart attack and death happen when the arteries become so narrow that blood is prevented from getting to the heart.

- **Type II diabetes**. As you read in Unit 5, insulin reduces the blood glucose level by making the liver and muscles take glucose from the blood and store it as glycogen. In type II diabetes, the body doesn't make enough insulin or it can't use the insulin it produces. As a result, blood glucose levels rise, which can damage blood vessels, nerves and organs. Type II diabetes runs in families, but people who are overweight or obese because they don't eat a healthy diet are also at risk of developing type II diabetes.

Links to Unit 5, pages 122 and 124.

Undernutrition

- **Kwashiorkor** is caused by a severe protein deficiency in very young children. It causes slow growth, exhaustion, oedema, diarrhoea and a swollen abdomen. It usually occurs in developing countries where parents are unable to feed their children a healthy, balanced diet because, for example, they can't afford to buy nutritious food, harvests fail, transport is poor, or war makes food unavailable.

**Good health
depends on a
nutritionally
balanced diet.**

remember

- **Marasmus** is the condition in which the muscle and fat of young children waste away. It occurs when breast milk or a weaning diet is low in nutrients, particularly protein and energy. It can lead to infections, dehydration and circulation disorders that can be fatal. Like kwashiorkor, it usually occurs in developing countries where people are unable to feed their children a healthy, balanced diet.

Nutritional deficiencies

www.food.gov.uk
www.nutrition.org.uk
www.vegsoc.org
www.eatwell.gov.uk/healthydiet
www.helptheaged.org.uk
www.nutrition.org.uk
www.mindbodysoul.gov.uk

Type II diabetes

Type II diabetes can occur in people whose diet contains too much glucose (sugar). Service users can reduce their blood glucose level by losing weight and eating a diet that:

Glycaemic index (GI)
A measure of how quickly carbohydrates are digested to release glucose into the blood.

- contains carbohydrates that have a low **glycaemic index (GI)**; low GI carbohydrates release glucose slowly into the blood, helping to maintain constant blood glucose levels

- is low in fat

- is high in fibre

- contains plenty of fruit and vegetables.

Lactose intolerance

Lactose is a sugar that is present in milk and dairy foods. It is sometimes added to foods such as meat products and baby foods. Some people have an intolerance to lactose. It causes them stomach cramps, wind and diarrhoea.

Service users who have lactose intolerance need to be careful with their diet. Packaged-food labels must be read to find out whether lactose has been added. Milk and dairy foods can be replaced by non-dairy products and soya milk. However, yoghurt doesn't usually cause many problems; neither do hard, mature cheeses, and cottage and cream cheese, because they only contain very small amounts of lactose.

Some service users are prescribed lactase enzyme, which is added to milk or taken as drops or capsules before eating. Lactase helps the digestion of lactose in a meal.

Food allergies

The word 'allergy' is used to describe a bad reaction by the body to an allergen. Allergens include pollen, dust mites, antibiotics and some foods. If your body reacts badly to a particular substance, you are said to be allergic to it. Anaphylaxis, or anaphylactic shock, is a whole-body allergic reaction and can be fatal.

Foods that cause allergies include milk, egg, wheat, soya, seafood, fruit and nuts. An allergic reaction to food usually happens quickly and symptoms include:

- itching and swelling of the mouth, lips, throat and skin

- vomiting and diarrhoea

- dizziness

- coughing and wheezing

- runny nose.

Menus and packaged food labels indicate whether food contains or is likely to contain allergens. Service users who have food allergies must avoid any food to which they are allergic and replace it with alternatives that ensure they don't miss out on essential nutrients.

Phenylketonuria (PKU)

Phenylalanine is an essential amino acid which the body needs to grow and work properly. However, too much phenylalanine can be harmful. PKU is an inherited condition in which phenylalanine builds up in the body, particularly in the brain where it causes severe and irreversible damage. The signs of PKU include:

- slow developmental and severe learning difficulties
- epilepsy
- eczema
- very fair hair
- musty smelling urine.

Service users who have PKU must eat a special low-phenylalanine diet. They must avoid meat and other protein-rich foods and eat 'safe', substitute proteins instead. Pregnant women who have PKU must follow the special diet or they risk miscarriage and brain damage in their baby, even if it hasn't inherited PKU.

Religious and cultural dietary requirements

Table 9.4 Dietary requirements of different religious and cultural groups

Religious/cultural group	Dietary requirements
Hindus	Hindus are not allowed to eat beef or drink alcohol. They rarely eat fish.
Jews	Jews are not allowed to eat pork or fish that doesn't have scales and fins. Any meat they eat must be kosher. In addition, meat and dairy foods must not be eaten together.
Muslims	Muslims are not allowed to eat pork or shellfish or to drink alcohol.
Vegetarians	Vegetarians don't eat meat and most don't eat fish. As you read earlier, it is important that they eat a varied diet to make sure they take in enough essential amino acids.
Vegans	Vegans don't eat any food that comes from animals. They must eat a wide selection of plant food to make sure they take in enough energy, essential amino acids, vitamins and minerals.

Links to Unit 4, pages 81–90.

Two-day plan

When planning a healthy diet (breakfast, midday and evening meals, snacks and beverages) for different individuals, there are a number of factors to take into consideration.

Figure 9.7
Planning for healthy eating

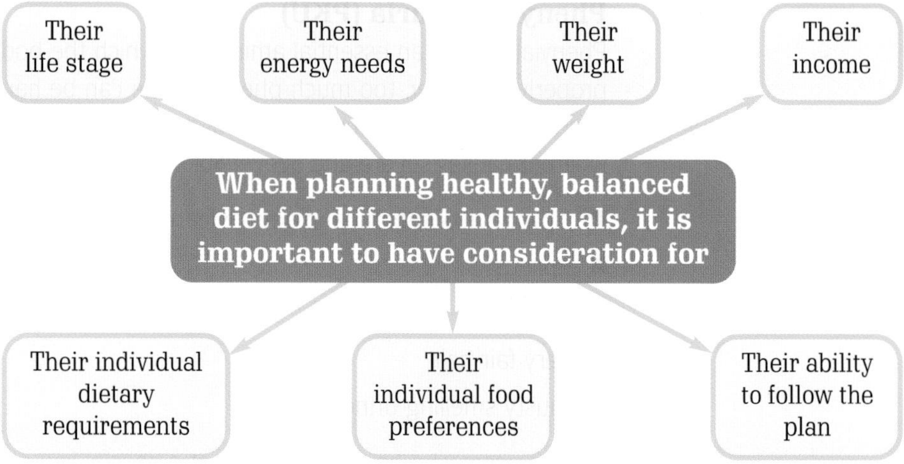

Their life stage

Their energy needs

Their weight

Their income

When planning healthy, balanced diet for different individuals, it is important to have consideration for

remember
We are all different and have different dietary needs.

Their individual dietary requirements

Their individual food preferences

Their ability to follow the plan

---

activity
INDIVIDUAL WORK (9.5)

P4

M3

D2

Use or copy the following table to demonstrate your understanding of dietary needs.

Table 9.5

Reason for special diet	How menus at my school, college or workplace cater for special dietary requirements	How the menus meet special dietary needs

---

case study
9.2

A two-day plan

Annie is 84 years old and obese. She is no longer able to shop and cook but care workers bring in food and make her meals. Yusef, a 25 year-old Muslim, is homeless and relies on shelters provided by charitable organisations for his meals. Kira is six years old and allergic to milk and nuts.

activity
GROUP WORK

(a) What affects the diets of Annie, Yusef and Kira?

(b) Produce a two-day diet plan for each individual. Make sure you cover breakfast, a midday and evening meal, snacks and beverages.

(c) Describe why Annie, Yusef and Kira require a different diet.

(d) Explain how your diet plans meet each person's needs.

www.bbc.co.uk/health

www.netdoctor.co.uk

www.nhsdirect.nhs.uk

www.weightwatchers.co.uk

www.weightlossresources.co.uk

www.diabetes.org.uk

www.bupa.org

www.nspku.org

www.ethnicityonline.net

The Principles of Food Safety and Hygiene

<table>
<tr><td>**keyword**</td><td>**Toxins**
Poisonous substances.</td></tr>
</table>

Food that is not stored and handled safely can become contaminated (spoiled) by bacteria or the **toxins** they produce, and by **pests**. If we eat food that has been contaminated, we run the risk of food poisoning. Vulnerable service users are most at risk of food poisoning. For this reason, it is essential that health and care workers follow safe practices when handling food.

Safe practices
Hygiene control

<table>
<tr><td>**keyword**</td><td>**Pests**
Animals that are hazardous to health, e.g. pets, flies, rats, mice, cockroaches and birds.</td></tr>
</table>

Food poisoning can be prevented by having high standards of hygiene. All health and care workers who are involved in the handling of food must:

- wash their hands with soap and water before handling food

- wash their hands with soap and water after:

  - using the toilet

  - helping service users use the toilet

  - handling raw food and rubbish

  - coughing, sneezing, using a handkerchief and touching their face or hair

- wear protective clothing

- keep their nails short and clean and their hair clean and tied back or covered

- not wear nail varnish or jewellery

- keep wounds covered with coloured waterproof dressings and check that they are allowed to handle food when wearing a dressing

- not smoke in a food area. It is against the law!

In addition, if they or anyone they live with is unwell, health and care workers must tell someone in authority at work. It may be that they will not be allowed to work with food for the time being.

The Impact of Diet on Health

To prevent the spread of bacteria from food and equipment:

- Cover and store raw and cooked foods in different fridges.
- If there is only one fridge, store raw foods on lower shelves than cooked foods.
- Use different work surfaces and equipment for raw and cooked foods.
- Keep work surfaces, equipment and wiping cloths thoroughly clean.
- Always serve food onto clean plates using clean utensils.

Figure 9.8
Hygiene control

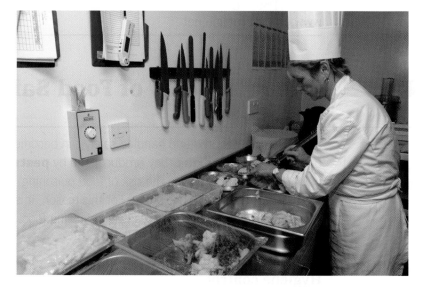

Temperature control

Food poisoning can be prevented by storing and cooking food at the right temperature:

- Store food according to the instructions on the packet, e.g. if it says 'Once opened, consume within three days' don't keep it for any longer!
- Refrigerate fresh food within two hours of purchase or preparation. Fridges must be kept at less than 5 °C.
- Freeze frozen food as quickly as possible after purchase. Freezers must be kept at less than −18 °C.
- Defrost frozen food in the fridge.
- Cook food according to the instructions on the packet.
- Use a food thermometer or a clean skewer to check that food is thoroughly cooked and piping hot before serving.
- If food has to be cooked in advance, cover it and keep it above 63 °C until it's time to eat.
- If food is microwaved, stir it from time to time to make sure it cooks evenly.

5 °C to 63 °C is the Temperature Danger Zone! Most bacteria thrive in the Temperature Danger Zone so store food below 5 °C or above 63 °C!

Pest control

Food poisoning can be prevented by controlling pests in food-storage and handling areas:

- Check for pests in storage, kitchen and eating areas and let your local Environmental Health Department know as soon as you see signs of an infestation, e.g. droppings.

- Throw out any food that might have been spoiled by pets or pests.

- Maintain a high standard of cleanliness – sweep floors, wipe up spills, wash and store equipment properly.

- Keep doors and windows closed, use fly screens.

- Keep food and waste covered and empty waste bins regularly.

Figure 9.9

Pests in food handling areas

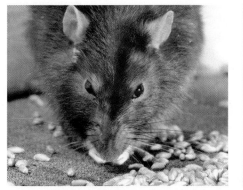
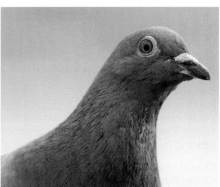
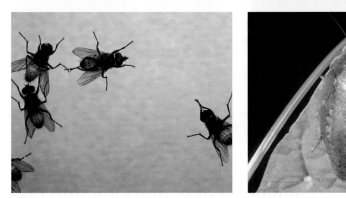

Effects of unsafe practices
Biological contamination of food

You read above that, if we eat food that is contaminated by bacteria or the toxins they produce, we are likely to get food poisoning. The table on page 212 describes the sources and symptoms of different types of food poisoning.

Chemical contamination of food

Chemicals such as washing-up liquid and bleach can contaminate food if they are not used carefully.

Physical contamination of food

Examples of physical contamination include:

- pieces of machinery that can fall into food when it is being manufactured
- bones, stones, pips, pieces of shell
- foreign objects, such as jewellery and pens, that can fall into food when it is being handled.

Table 9.6 Sources and symptoms of food poisoning

Source of food poisoning	Symptoms of food poisoning
Salmonella Salmonella is a bacterium usually found in the faeces of infected people and animals and in poultry, eggs, meat and water.	■ abdominal pain, watery and bloody diarrhoea or constipation ■ headaches ■ nausea and vomiting ■ fever
Campylobacter Campylobacter is a bacterium usually found in undercooked meat (especially poultry), unpasteurised milk and untreated water.	■ severe diarrhoea and abdominal pain ■ blood in the faeces
Bacillus cereus Bacillus cereus is a bacterium found mainly in rice dishes and sometimes in pasta, meat or vegetable dishes, dairy products, soups, sauces and sweet pastry products. It is also found in the soil and in dust.	■ diarrhoea and abdominal pain ■ nausea and vomiting
Clostridium perfringens Clostridium perfringens is a bacterium that occurs naturally in the intestine in people and animals, in the soil and in dust.	■ diarrhoea and abdominal pain
Escherichia coli E. coli is a bacterium that occurs naturally in the intestines of people and animals. Most types of E. coli don't cause illness but some release toxins that contaminate food or water.	■ stomach cramps and diarrhoea ■ vomiting ■ blood in the faeces
Staphylococcus aureus Staph aureus is a bacterium found in the nose, throat, in boils and in pus. Like E. coli, it produces a toxin that contaminates both cooked food, e.g. meat, and prepared food, e.g. cream.	■ diarrhoea and abdominal pain ■ severe vomiting

Legislation, regulations and codes of practice

Workplaces have health and safety policies that are based on food safety legislation and regulations. Health and safety codes of practice (procedures) tell workers how to do their job in ways that comply with legislation and regulations and, more importantly, promote the health and safety of service users. They include:

remember

Safe food-handling practices are key to good health.

- hygiene and food-safety procedures, which describe safe and hygienic food-handling methods and which protect against food poisoning
- infection control procedures, which describe how to work with service users who have food poisoning and who to report incidences of food poisoning to.

Figure 9.10

Legislation, regulations and codes of practice that ensure food safety and hygiene

The Food Safety Act 1990
This act is particularly relevant to anyone working in the food safety industry. It aims to ensure that all food produced for sale is safe to eat, reaches quality expectations and is not misleadingly presented

Food Hygiene Regulations 2006
These regulations apply to all food businesses. Their aim is to improve food safety and help reduce the number of cases of food poisoning

Legislation and regulations that ensure food safety and hygiene

Hazard Analysis Critical Control Point
HACCP is an internationally recognised and recommended system of food safety management. It identifies the 'critical points' in a process where food safety hazards could occur and puts steps in place to prevent things going wrong. This is sometimes referred to as 'controlling hazards'

Food Safety (Temperature Control) Regulations 1995
These regulations apply to all food businesses. They require that food must not be kept at a temperature that will allow the growth of bacteria or the formation of toxins that cause ill health

activity
GROUP WORK (9.6)

P5

M4

(a) Carry out a survey of the kitchen at your school, college or workplace and identify the safe practices used when preparing, cooking and serving food.

(b) Produce a PowerPoint presentation that describes why these safe practices are necessary.

i

www.food.gov.uk
www.healthpromotionagency.org.uk
www.foodlink.org.uk
www.hpa.org.uk/infections
http://nursing.about.com/od/patienteducation

1. What particular nutrients make up a balanced diet?

2. Explain the importance of each of these.

3. What particular nutrients are important for an infant, a child, an adolescent, an adult, a pregnant woman, a woman who is breastfeeding and an elderly person?

4. Describe the factors that influence what you eat.

5. Describe two medical conditions that result from not eating a balanced diet.

6. Explain why the dietary needs of people experiencing these two medical conditions are different.

7. Explain, with examples, why it is necessary to use safe practices when preparing, cooking and handling food.

Books

Blades, M. (2004), *Intermediate Nutrition and Health* (Highfield Publications)

Food Standards Agency (2005), *Manual of Nutrition* (The Stationery Office Books)

Hudson, P. and Symonds, C. (1996), *Nutrition and Hygiene for Caterers* (Hodder Arnold)

Mackean, D. G. (1988), *Human Life* (John Murray)

Mackean, D. G. and Jones, B. (1987), *Introduction to Human and Social Biology* (John Murray)

Minett, P., Wayne, D. and Rubenstein, D. (1999), *Health Sciences* (Collins Educational)

Page, M. (ed) (2005), *The Human Body* (Dorling Kindersley)

Sprenger, R. (2001), *The Essentials of Food Hygiene* (Highfield Publications)

Sprenger, R. (2002), *The Essentials of Food Safety: a Guide for Carers* (Highfield Publications)

Sprenger, R. (2005), *The Food Hygiene Handbook* (Highfield Publications)

Windsor, G. and Moonie, N. (ed) (2000), *GNVQ Health and Social Care: Intermediate Compulsory Units with Edexcel Options* (Heinemann)

Wright, D. (2000), *Human Physiology and Health* (Heinemann)

Wright, D. (2001), *Human Physiology and Health for GCSE: Resource Pack* (Heinemann)

Glossary

Align – Line up or make straight.

Anatomy – The structure of the body, i.e. the way different parts of the body are put together.

Anus – The opening in a person's bottom through which faeces (waste material) is excreted from the body.

Atheroma – A thick, fatty sludge which forms plaques on artery walls, reducing the space through which blood can flow.

Autism – A disorder in which people are unable to interact with others.

Ayurvedic medicine – A system of diet, exercise, meditation and herbal remedies that is used to treat imbalances in the body.

Body system – A group of organs working together to carry out one or more functions.

Career development plan – An action plan that shows how you aim to move forward in your career.

Charter – A description of an organisation's purpose.

Code of conduct – The standards which govern how people behave.

Code of practice – A set of rules.

Community cohesion – Development of good relationships and equal opportunities between people from different backgrounds at work and in schools and neighbourhoods.

Continence – Control of the bladder and bowel.

Cooperation – Teamwork, collaboration.

Coronary arteries – Blood vessels that supply the heart muscle with blood.

Cross infection – Passing of an infection from one person to another.

Decentralisation – Spread of control of services from central government to local government.

Dementia – A condition which causes memory loss, confusion and loss of mental ability and social skills.

Deprived – Disadvantaged, underprivileged.

Develop – Become more complex.

Diet – The food we eat on a day-to-day basis.

Glossary

Norms of behaviour – The way society expects us to behave in different situations.

Obesity – An excessive amount of body fat.

Online – Using the Internet.

Oppression – Harsh, cruel treatment.

Orthodox – Keeping to traditional teachings and beliefs.

Palliative care – Care which aims to kill pain.

Peer pressure – Pressure from one's peers to behave in a way that is similar to or acceptable by them.

Peers – People in the same age group, social group, etc.

Personal skills – Behaviours that are part of our personalities.

Pests – Animals that are hazardous to health, e.g. pets, flies, rats, mice, cockroaches and birds.

Physiology – The function of the body, i.e. the way different parts of the body work, both on their own and together.

Policy – An official document that describes how an organisation aims to carry out its business.

Pressure ulcers – Wounds caused by pressure or friction.

Probationary period – The period of time during which a new member of staff is monitored to see if they and the job are right for each other.

Procedure – A way of doing things.

Proofread – Read a piece of writing to check for mistakes.

Qualification frameworks – A set of qualifications at different levels.

Reaction time – The time it takes for someone to respond to a stimulus or change in the situation.

Reminiscence – Looking back, remembering.

Repetitive strain injuries – Injuries caused by repeating movements over and over again.

Responsibility – The duties or tasks that are part of the job role, e.g. hoovering, dusting, washing windows.

Role model – Someone we copy because we respect and admire them.

Self-confidence – To be confident in your own abilities.

Self-esteem – To have a good opinion about yourself.

Self-refer – To choose for yourself to visit your GP, dentist, etc.

Self-respect – To feel you behave in an admirable and correct way.

Service providers – Organisations that meet the needs of the public.

Service user groups – Groups of people who have similar care needs, such as children, elderly people, people with sensory impairments and people with learning difficulties.

Service users – People that health and social care services help. They include patients and social care clients and their friends, families and carers.

Sharps – Hazardous sharp equipment such as needles, scalpel blades, scissors, razors and lancets.

Siblings – Brothers and sisters.

Signer – Somebody who translates speech into signs that can be understood by people with a hearing impairment.

Signs – The visible marks of an illness, e.g. swollen glands.

Skills – Things you are good at doing, e.g. swimming, cooking.

Social exclusion – Being left out, not allowed to join in.

Social role – The part people play in their family, community, at school and work, etc.

Social skills – Behaviours we need in order to socialise successfully with other people.

Socialisation – The process of rearing children to think and behave in the ways that their family and society expects of them.

Status – Position compared with others, e.g. sister, manager, chief inspector.

Symptoms – The feelings that accompany an illness, e.g. a headache.

Therapeutic – Healing.

Toxins – Poisonous substances.

Translator – Someone who can express the meaning of words and expressions in another language.

Tsunami – A long, high sea wave caused by an underwater earthquake.

Unprotected sex – Having sex without using any contraception, which may lead to pregnancy or catching a sexually transmitted infection.

Vegans – People who don't eat meat and animal products, such as milk and eggs.

Work–life balance – A healthy balance between work time and personal time.

Index

Page numbers in italics *indicate* figures or tables.

Index

menopause *130*
mental health care needs 146
messages, misinterpreting 12
minerals *198*
movement therapy 153
multi-agency working 181, *182*
musculoskeletal system 114
music therapy 152–3
Muslims 86–7

nannies 188
National Health Service (NHS) 18, 173, 174, 175
needs of individuals 29–32
    care needs 143–7, *144*, 156–7
    factors influencing 33–44
nervous system 112
night blindness *204*
non-verbal communication 5, *5*, 160–1
nursery nurses 189
nurses 190
nursing assistants 189
nutrients 197, *198*, *204*

obesity 202, 205, *205*
observations, routine 120–1
old age
    care needs *144*, 145
    development during *130*, *131*, *132*
    diet during 199
organs of the body 107–10, *107*
ovaries 110, *113*

paganism 87–8
pancreas 109, *113*
parathyroid gland *113*
parenthood 138
partnership working 181–5
PCTs (Primary Care Trusts) 174, *174*, 183
peak flow 119–20
personal hygiene 38–9
personal space 67
pest control and food safety 211
phenylketonuria (PKU) 207
physical abuse 43
physical growth and development 129, *130*
physical needs 30, 143–4, *144*, 146–7, 156–7
pituitary gland *113*
playgroups 176
policies 17, 70
pollution 35
prejudice 19, *19*
Primary Care Trusts (PCTs) 174, *174*, 183
primary health care 174
privacy, respecting 23
private organisations 65, 173

procedures 17, 70
proteins *198*
proximity 67
puberty *130*, *131*
pulse rate 118

Rastafarianism 88
receptionists 188
redundancy 139
religion
    dietary requirements *207*
    different beliefs 81–90
    and equality of opportunity *91*
    and health and needs 38
reminiscence therapy 153
Reporting of Injuries, Diseases and Dangerous Occurrences Regulations (RIDDOR) 167
reproductive system 113–14
resources 69–70, *69*, 185
respect, showing during care 146
respiratory system 111–12
retirement 139
rheumatoid arthritis (RA) 125
rickets *204*
rights, individual 21–3
    and Care Value Base 23–4
    protecting 23–6, 97–100, *97*, *98*, *100*
role play 152

salmonella 212
schools 176–7
    starting school 137
scurvy *204*
secondary health care 174–5, *175*
security 50–1
self-actualisation 30
self-concept 140–2
self-confidence 30, 31
self-esteem 30, 31, 32, 141, 161, *162*
self-harm 43
self-image 140–1, *140*, 141
self-respect 30
sensory impairment
    care needs 144–5
    and communication 9, *9*, 10
service users 2
    care needs 125–6, 156–7
    creative/therapeutic activities for 151–68
    involvement of 182
    protecting rights of 97, *97*, 99, 100, *100*
specific dietary needs 205–7, *207*
services see health and social care services
settings
    for creative/therapeutic activities *151*
    for health and social care 176–9
sex (male or female) 79
sexual abuse 44